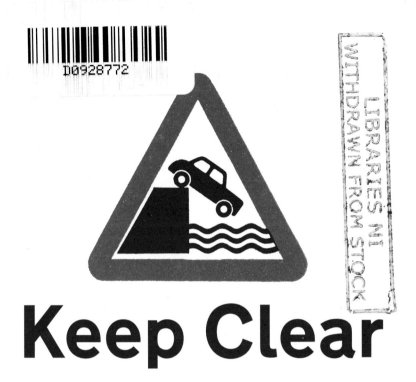

Keep Clear

My adventures with Asperger's

Tom Cutler

SCRIBE

Melbourne • London

Scribe Publications

2 John St, Clerkenwell, London, WC1N 2ES, United Kingdom

18–20 Edward St, Brunswick, Victoria 3056, Australia

Published by Scribe in 2019

The Autism-Spectrum Quotient and empathising–systemising
(E–S) theory scatter plot have been reproduced in this book by kind
permission of the Autism Research Centre.

Typeset in Bembo by the publishers

Printed and bound in the UK by CPI Group (UK) Ltd, Croydon,
CR0 4YY

9781911617563 (UK edition)

9781925713770 (Australian edition)

9781925693157 (e-book)

Catalogue records for this book are available from the National
Library of Australia and the British Library.

scribepublications.co.uk

scribepublications.com.au

For Marianne

Then said they unto him, Say now Shibboleth:
and he said Sibboleth: for he could not
frame to pronounce *it* right.

JUDGES 12:6

Contents

Prologue

On the desk in front of me, bearing the crown and shield of the royal coat of arms of Her Majesty's Stationery Office, is Statutory Instrument Number 1857, *The Traffic Signs Regulations and General Directions 1964*. This document sets out the now familiar system of signage devised for use on British roads after 1 January 1965. The floppy 112-page compendium contains specimen signs set in the attractive and superbly efficient Transport typeface — *Ring road*, *Picnic area*, *Cattle grid* — alongside rules for the deployment of Britain's classic pictographic road signs — red circles and triangles containing a cow, falling rocks, a walking man, each pared down to its quintessential silhouette.

The booklet gives off a musty, friendly smell. It is the smell of years on an antiquarian bookseller's shelf, the smell of 1964. Circling the government shield, a heraldic garter bears the motto, *Honi soit qui mal y pense*, 'Shame be on him that evil thinks', the maxim of a more polite, more trusting dominion now vanished. I love this little book and come back to it often.

On the shelf beyond are some of the other books that I return to time and again: *The Secrets of Conjuring and Magic*, 1877, by Jean Eugène Robert-Houdin; *An Essay on Typography* by Eric Gill; *Metro Maps of the World*; *The Oxford Medical Dictionary*. Non-fiction reference books all, these volumes highlight something of my eccentric and peculiar nature, which until lately had mystified and grieved me.

Why these weird interests? Why my strange tastes in music, food, and clothes, my persistent routines and loathing of variation? Why the hypersensitivity to sounds and smells, the mind-scrambling overload when in a supermarket or using a ticket machine? Why the crippling anguish when meeting people — and why had someone just told me, yet again, 'You are the rudest man I have ever met'?

For half a century, all this had been a painful puzzle, causing me frustration, bemusement, and deep loneliness. For decades, the real me had been hidden behind a façade of facile wit and practised social formulas. I was going through the motions.

That was until one night, not so long ago, when, the pressure inside me having built to an uncontainable degree, the floodgates burst in a brief episode of craziness.

Since that mini collapse, I have begun, little by little, and with the help of some expert people, to understand what's been going on for so long, to put a name to the shadows in the cave, to reconcile myself with myself.

The things that happen in this book are true, though various people and places have been disguised. But to understand how it all unfolded we must go back to the chilly autumn of 2015.

Chapter 1:
Falling rocks

Even in our sleep, pain, which cannot forget,
falls drop by drop upon the heart.

AESCHYLUS

It was four thirty on a dark September morning and I was suddenly
awake. I knew straight away that something was wrong.

The house was quiet and I could hear the steady breathing of
my wife Lea in bed beside me, but I was feeling extremely strange.
My pulse was pounding fast and hard, and with each beat my heart
seemed to strike my ribcage an abnormally hefty thump. I felt hot
and cold all over, my skin was prickling, and I was sweating like a
runner.

Outside, the street was dark and still, the hush disturbed only by the mewing of an early gull. The streetlamp opposite cast an eerie glow through the blinds and across my hands as I turned them over and over, closely examining the veins, which appeared black against the orange skin. Somehow they didn't seem to belong to me. Were they really different in some way or was the streetlight playing tricks? I took a hard look at my palms, crisscrossed as they are with the fine creases of middle age. Extending my arms in the semi-darkness I detected a growing tremor in my fingers. I was feeling very strange and very unwell. What the hell was this?

Sitting up, I swung my legs gingerly over the edge of the bed and planted my feet on the rug. Immediately below my ribcage my abdomen felt bloated. Did it look abnormal? By the green glimmer of the clock on the bedside table it was hard to say. One funny thing — my feet seemed to be more distant than they ought to be, as if seen through novelty glasses.

The periphery of my visual field began to narrow like a closing velvet pouch. I started to salivate. The area postrema, the so-called 'vomit centre' of the brain, was going into action. Feeling as if I might pass out, I tilted my torso sharply forward.

After a while, the nausea ebbed and I sat up again. My tremor had become a steady shiver now. I took a draught of water, holding on to the glass with both hands. All at once something very bad happened: I was overtaken by the alarming conviction that I was about to die. The sensation was real and frightening. This was it. I was going to die.

This sense of impending doom was something I remembered reading about. People having heart attacks sometimes report it. My own heart was now jumping spasmodically and my breathing was short and fast.

Was I having a heart attack? I know the symptoms because health is a subject in which I take a special interest. To Lea, it is actually more of an obsession. She says it's morbid to pore over the medical news every day, but I am fascinated by the mechanics of the body's processes and systems. I am a natural diagnostician, and perhaps would have made a good doctor. I remember as a boy being distracted by the back copies of *Nursing Mirror* in the reference library when I was supposed to be revising for my A levels. I would flip compulsively to the photographic quiz that illustrated distempers of every kind in harsh black-and-white, and would try to guess the disease, when I should have been going over my art history notes.

The typical symptoms of a heart attack include these:

1. Pain, pressure, or tightness in the centre of the chest, possibly travelling to the arm/s, jaw, neck, back, or abdomen
2. Lightheadedness or dizziness
3. Sweating
4. Shortness of breath
5. Nausea
6. A sense of imminent catastrophe
7. Coughing or wheezing

I hadn't got the main one, which is pain, and neither was I coughing or wheezing, but I did have numbers 2, 3, 4, 5, and 6. I looked at the clock. It said 4:33am. If this was a heart attack, I mustn't delay: time is muscle.

The first thing to do was call an ambulance. Then I should chew an aspirin to help bust any clots blocking the cardiac vessels.

With a shaky hand I picked up my phone, but with no chest

pain this frightening disturbance was probably not a heart attack. If it wasn't, an ambulance would be superfluous. I put the phone down again. The aspirin was likewise academic. Still, I might as well chew one. It couldn't do any harm.

This unemotional analysis was being done by the rational bit of my brain, watching me askance, as always, from slightly beside my left temple. Or so it seemed to me in my unhinged condition. Whatever this attack was, my autonomic nervous system was still in the throes of it. My hands were wet, my breathing rapid. I continued to shake.

I don't express emotion on the whole, but now tears began running down my nose, mingling with the rivulets of sweat. I knew that I was very ill, and I was frightened. I shook my wife's arm.

'Lea! Lea!' I gasped, trying to master my emotions, 'I think there's something wrong with me. Something's seriously wrong.'

Lea woke up and listened to me calmly. She is a positive, cheerful person, unlike me. I am cool, precise, ironic, a watcher in the shadows, prone to low moods and restlessness. Lea continued to look at me. I sat there quivering and gasping.

'What is it, Tom?'

'I think there's something terribly wrong,' I gulped.

She considered for a moment. Then she said, matter-of-factly, 'You're having a panic attack.'

Panic attack? Me? Don't be ridiculous. I've never had a panic attack. A panic attack is something other people have, not me. But in the turmoil the analytical bit of my brain took charge. I knew the symptoms of a panic attack:

1. Trembling
2. Rapid breathing

3. A feeling of impending doom
4. Racing heart or palpitations
5. Hot and cold flushes
6. Pins-and-needles
7. Lightheadedness
8. Sweating
9. Nausea
10. Tearfulness
11. Feelings of unreality or detachment

I had the lot, including number 11. Now I understood the strange idea that my hands were not my own. 'Yes,' I said to myself. 'These are the symptoms of a panic attack.' But my body wasn't impressed by the diagnosis and went on trembling and sweating.

If you are hiking in the Rocky Mountains and come unexpectedly face to face with a grizzly bear, an aspect of your brain called the limbic system will come into its own. This primitive so-called 'lizard brain' is responsible for the 'four Fs', which are, in the words of one witty biologist, feeding, fighting, fleeing, and mating.

In the fight-or-flight response to danger, the brain causes the release of hormones that help the body to run away or fight. These hormones include cortisol and most significantly adrenaline. Adrenaline increases the heart rate and blood pressure, makes you sweat and tremble, and gives you a dry mouth. Cortisol puts your blood glucose up. Now your alertness is heightened, and as the body tries to take in more oxygen to feed its muscles your breathing quickens. Because blood is being diverted from the brain to more immediately critical parts, you can become lightheaded and nauseous.

An entirely imaginary or unrealistic threat occasioned by some nameless fear will provoke the same responses as a real bear. If you have ever delivered a speech to an audience you will understand how the fight-or-flight response can make you feel even when you are in no immediate physical danger. You will probably get a dry mouth, become very alert, and experience a strong desire to run away.

'Would you like a cup of tea?' asked Lea.

I nodded and she went downstairs to make one.

I wiped my hand over my face then put it to my chest. The old heart was banging away but there was still no pain and my sixth sense was telling me that, yes, this was a head problem not a heart problem.

Shortly I heard the stair creak as Lea returned with the tea. It was pale and weak-looking. Why must I always be so critical?

'Thanks,' I whispered.

My breathing was slowing, the vagus nerve cranking the parasympathetic nervous system into gear, gradually bringing things back into balance.

I went and splashed water on my face. There was a lot more salt than pepper in that stubble these days. I looked tired, too.

As I padded back into the bedroom, Lea peered at me expectantly: 'Okay?'

I couldn't decide. Was this really a panic attack? If so, what had caused it and how could I find out? I needed some answers because I didn't ever want another one of those, thank you very much.

★

The roots of mental distress are, of course, not always obvious. Our subconscious mind seems able to go to great lengths to hide such origins from us. For some time, I had been troubled by bad nightmares, which woke me up or made me shout out in my sleep. In the most recent one, I had thought Lea was creeping in to strangle me with the cord of her dressing gown as I slept. I cried out, and so vivid was the picture that, as she tried to calm me down, I thought the dream was coming true. Five thirty in the morning is no time to be wrestling with a thrashing husband when you've got a busy day ahead of you.

I had been waking at an ungodly hour for quite a while, lying there, staring at the ceiling, turning things over in my mind. I recognised early waking as a classic symptom of depression, and it was true that my mood had been low for ages. From a golden sunset to a good meal, I found life unrewarding. My hobbies had lapsed: typography, sleight-of-hand magic, and British road signage had been the focus of my interest for a long time, but now they disgusted me a bit.

I remembered F. Scott Fitzgerald's account of his own troubles in 'The Crack-Up':

> I had weaned myself from all the things I used to love
> … every act of life from the morning toothbrush to the
> friend at dinner had become an effort. I saw that for a
> long time I had not liked people and things, but only
> followed the rickety old pretense of liking.

I was touchy and irritable, unable to read the papers or listen to the news without shouting at the radio. After dinner, I would pace the room, driving Lea to distraction. Family friends found me hard work. During one pub lunch, after I'd wolfed a sandwich and a lemonade as the other three laughed and chatted over their roast beef and beer, one of them asked me sharply, 'Why do you never *savour* a meal?' My distant social disposition was damaging friendships.

Yet I was happily married, I was fairly healthy, and some of my books had spent time on bestseller lists around the world. So why the constant knot in my stomach?

I stopped ruminating and had a last mouthful of tea. It was tepid. Lea told me to try to sleep. She was probably more concerned than she let on. I managed to doze unsteadily till dawn.

In the morning I made an appointment to see the duty doctor at the walk-in clinic. I got an early slot, so the waiting room was not full. On the board was an announcement about blood pressure. I noticed that the heading, which was in capitals, had not been letterspaced. This irritated me beyond endurance and I had to move to a chair where I couldn't see the offending paper. As Jan Tschichold, the great typographer, famously pointed out, 'Words in capitals must always be letterspaced. The spacing of the capitals in lines of importance should be very carefully optically equalized.' Surely people knew this? Or maybe they didn't. What other people think or know has long been a puzzle to me.

My deliberation was interrupted by a crackly command from the wall-speaker calling me in to see Dr Sam.

I sat down perpendicular to the doctor.

'So how are you, Tom?'

Sir William Osler, the so-called 'father of modern medicine', coined a useful adage for student doctors: 'Just listen to your patient, he is telling you the diagnosis.' Taking a leaf from his book, Dr Sam was using the classic open question designed to get the patient to spill the beans.

'Well,' I said, 'I'm worried there might be something seriously wrong with me. My stomach seems bloated — I just don't feel right.'

After examining me, Dr Sam gave me a searching look. 'I can't find anything physically wrong. There's no swelling that I can feel, but we'll run some tests, just to be sure. If I might say so, you do seem rather tense …'

I didn't know it, but I'd struck lucky; Dr Sam had trained at the Maudsley psychiatric hospital.

'I've been feeling bad for some time,' I confessed. 'I can't seem to enjoy things any more.'

The doctor nodded. 'What you're describing is called "anhedonia". It's a kind of depression in which you are unable to take an interest in or get pleasure from normally enjoyable activities.'

She observed me ambiguously. Was it my turn to say something?

'I don't really know how I feel,' I said. 'Sort of "empty". I'm finding social situations increasingly hard.'

'We think the zestlessness you've described has something to do with the brain's reward system. Something might be wrong with your dopamine levels. But first we need to find out what's causing the depression and do something about that.'

Now seemed the right time to tell her about the other thing.

'I've had what my wife thinks might have been a panic attack,' I said, guardedly.

'Are you an anxious person, would you say?'

I hadn't really ever thought of myself as anxious — low mood, yes, but anxious people wrung their hands, jumped at noises, worried about everything, and suffered from what used to be called 'their nerves'. I considered the idea. Maybe it would explain the constant tightness in my chest, the endless pacing up and down, my suppressed rage at a friend's one-minute-late arrival for lunch.

'I suppose I could be described as anxious, yes,' I said, putting my answer in the passive voice so as to distance myself as far as possible from responsibility.

'What makes you anxious?'

'Being alive in the world,' I replied. I got a genuine laugh in response. This is how I deflect threats, but I meant it. I'm sometimes accused of not taking things seriously. The opposite is true.

'Does anything in particular make you anxious?' asked Dr Sam.

'Other people,' I said.

No laugh. She was obviously rationed to one laugh per patient per appointment. Through the window I watched a small plane, which had just taken off from the airport, climbing silently over the river.

'The ugly sisters of anxiety and depression are related,' she explained, revolving a pencil between her fingers. 'But they're not the same thing. Panic attacks are a symptom of anxiety. They usually happen during the day, but they can also come at nighttime and wake you up. Because of the anxiety your brain is unusually alert, so it construes minor nocturnal changes in your body as signs of threat.'

The blue polymer mattress on which I'd been examined was covered with a sheet of papery material that had been creased as I got off it. I had a powerful urge to get up and smooth it out.

Dr Sam explained that there were things we could try for the low mood and the anxiety. There were antidepressants, but these might have side effects. We'd leave pills till we'd tried other options.

She looked at me over her glasses. 'Do you know what cognitive behavioural therapy is?'

My heart sank. 'Yes,' I said. I knew CBT was a common and supposedly successful 'talking therapy'.

'Would you be willing to try that?'

I saw myself standing alone at the top of a hill, surveying a landscape of green meadows and chocolate-box cottages. Birds sang in the trees and dopamine flowed in tranquil streams, cheering the butterflies amongst the tussocks.

'Would you be happy to try that?' repeated Dr Sam.

I attempted to give the impression that I had been pondering the matter. 'I'll give it a go,' I said. It seemed churlish to say no.

'There is a waiting list of a few weeks to see a therapist, but I could refer you to an online CBT programme called SunBurst while you're waiting to see a real live person. How does that sound?'

'Online? It sounds implausible,' I said ungratefully, 'and commercial. But I'm miserable enough to try anything.'

And so I was sent on my way and told to stand by for news from the SunBurst people. I left the doctor's and walked past the building-site where they are tearing down the hospital in which my son was born and putting up some new flats. I crossed the road by the old Red Lion, now a Tesco store with reversing lorries, and made my way back home along the edge of the park, where some children were chasing a pigeon with a bad foot.

I live in an old shipbuilding port on the south coast of England, and a sea fret was beginning to roll in over the town. Now and again, the low moan of a foghorn could be heard across the harbour. As I headed down towards the church at the end of my road, I noticed that the top of the tower was veiled in mist.

My way took me through the church yard, and I stopped as I sometimes do to look at the graves. I found myself at the burial place of Master Mariner Thomas Boyce, who died on 9 September 1881, aged 55. Disconcertingly, this was my own age. The grave was surmounted by an unusual stone. Carved into the shape of a pitched roof, it hugged the ground, its once bright masonry now grey and lichen-blotched. Twisted ropes snaked along its ridge and around the chiselled anchor that leant against its 'gable end'. In lead:

ERECTED BY DANIEL DE PASS IN TESTIMONY OF HIS APPRECI-
ATION OF THE UPRIGHT CHARACTER AND VALUED SERVICES
OF CAPTAIN BOYCE DURING THE 33 YEARS HE WAS IN THE
EMPLOY OF DE PASS & CO. OF CAPE TOWN.

What, I wondered, had the upright Thomas Boyce known of anxiety?

I wandered home, shut the door, and hung up my coat. I noticed that my bloated feeling had faded away. It had been worrying me for days but now it was gone. I thought about Dr Sam and her diagnosis. Was there something in it? In this age of instant news and instant noodles, so-called 'talking therapy' was surely nothing but the latest flavour of the month, wasn't it? It wouldn't help me to find out what was really needling me, would it? It was going to be a waste of everybody's time. After the excitements of the night it all seemed a bit of a let-down.

But without my knowing it, something had already started to happen. Before long, a new light would be faded up on the dark backstage of my character and, with a bit of help, I would come to see that my panic attack had been long primed to explode. I was going to uncover the mystery of just what it was that for years had been souring my relationships; getting me into scrapes; winding my spring.

I put the kettle on.

★

Days passed; the sun came out; the rain came down. I remained steadily grey. Every morning I brushed my teeth. Every evening I brushed them again. Up and down. Up and down. Every Tuesday the bell ringers practised: a soothing sound. Lea was busy at work. Now and again I caught her looking at me. While I was waiting to hear from SunBurst I thought I would walk along to the library and read up on anxiety.

The word itself has been around since the early sixteenth century, but its use in English has become steadily more common since the 1960s. It comes from the Latin *anxius* (choke) and is related to *angere* (to torment), which is a parent also to 'anger', 'anguish', and 'angst', three other emotions with which I was familiar.

The definition of 'anxiety' in Oxford's online dictionary is, 'A feeling of worry, nervousness, or unease, typically about an imminent event or something with an uncertain outcome.' If this was true, it wasn't quite what I had. My unease was with me from the moment I woke up. There was no imminent event with an uncertain outcome. It was chronic.

Psychiatrists see anxiety as a nervous disorder characterised by excessive apprehension — not so much a condition in itself as a symptom of several other ailments. It comes in a variety of flavours, each of which expresses the feelings of inner turmoil in a different way. I flipped through the list I had made.

First on the cards was post-traumatic stress disorder. PTSD arises after a person has experienced a very frightening or dangerous crisis, such as a bad car crash, a violent personal attack, or military combat. This didn't sound like me.

Next was a common form of anxiety called social anxiety disorder, or 'social phobia'. A dread of social situations, more pronounced than shyness, it is an intense irrational fear of mixing with people or even of speaking on the phone. This struck a chord. I recalled something that I had forgotten from my early years, when I worked in publishing.

From time to time as a young man, while making a routine phone call to a print supplier, I would suddenly be struck dumb, unable to get out any sound beyond a croak. Frightened and embarrassed, I would replace the receiver and sit quiet for a few minutes to allow my trembling to subside. I couldn't understand what was going on. The people I was speaking to were friendly, and in the unwritten social hierarchy of business relationships when I said 'Jump!' they were supposed to ask 'How high?' It was just that, for a reason I couldn't grasp, I sometimes found the experience of speaking to them on the phone grossly threatening. It always came out of the blue and it was always inexplicable and alarming. Once I had recovered from each puzzling episode, however, I paid it little attention, and over time I allowed myself to 'forget' that anything had ever happened.

For as long as I could recall, parties had also been difficult for me, provoking silent dread days ahead. I vividly remember at my own seventh birthday party watching the other children playing games and having fun, while I stood uncomprehending and resentful at the edge, with an invisible forcefield somehow separating me from them, unable to break in.

By the time I was being invited to parties during my teenage years — an infrequent occurrence — I had learned to pre-medicate myself with alcohol. I knew that a bottle of beer fifteen minutes before any kind of social gathering was enough to blunt the fear and make me more able to join in. Two bottles was even better.

In 2016, a team from University Hospital in Basel decided to test what everybody thought they already knew: that booze is a good social lubricant. They gave sixty healthy men and women a glass of beer each, either alcoholic or non-alcoholic. Then they waited. After a while, they administered mood and empathy tests to both groups.

The results were interesting. The desire to be with others in a happy, chatty, and open environment was greater in the alcohol group than in the non-alcohol group, but the effect was stronger in those who had shown higher social inhibitions to start off with. The alcohol drinkers were also quicker than the non-alcohol drinkers to recognise happiness among a variety of facial expressions, and they displayed more emotional empathy, particularly if they had shown less of it at the beginning.

These findings might explain why many anxious people drink alcohol, and why so many of them get into trouble with it.

Alcohol is a depressant which, paradoxically, makes you more lively and less anxious. But though it can oil the social wheels, it is a hard drug to manage because as well as relaxing your nerves it will also depress your vigilance so that you end up having too much. The American humorist James Thurber put it in a nutshell: 'One is all right, two is too many, three is not enough.'

I mentally ticked the *social anxiety* box. This one was spot on. They were talking about me.

Another common complaint on the list was generalised anxiety disorder (GAD). GAD sufferers have an imbalance of mood regulators such as adrenaline and serotonin. They are anxious most of the time about a whole range of things, and often cannot remember when they last felt relaxed. Restless and worrisome, they suffer insomnia and palpitations. Should one anxiety pass, another is likely to take its place.

Here again was a condition I recognised.

All this was quite a surprise, not to say a revelation. Within a short time I had gone from being a man who was feeling a bit low, who believed anxiety to be a complaint of the fey, jumpy, and nervous, to being a classic case, having not one but two of the items on the menu.

Generalised anxiety disorder was, I learned, more likely to occur in those who have a close relative with the same thing, and this made me think. I wondered whether the anxiety, which I now recognised as a longstanding part of my makeup, might be inherited.

I thought about my parents and remembered my father at the seaside, when I was a boy. He would stand at the water's edge as his children splashed about, watching us like a lifeguard. Every now and then he would shout an angry warning about the deadly dangers all around us. He was incredibly tense. At night if anyone got up to use the loo he would call out 'Who's that?!', and walking across a bridge over the bypass his heart would race so much that he was prescribed pills. When my mother recently forgot to ring him from a family do that she had driven to, he paced up and down, beside himself with vague terror.

My mother herself is a tremendously anxious woman who will tremble and cry if one of her grown-up children is a few minutes late for a lunch appointment. I recall her telling me that the over-whelming atmosphere in her household as she was growing up was one of anxiety, which emanated, she said, from her own mother.

I don't remember my grandmother as anxious. A Victorian lady of rather censorious demeanour, she seemed merely dour, terse, and aloof. Little did I then know that this is just how many people see me. Maybe it *was* in the genes.

There was plenty to get through on the subject of anxiety, but after a couple of weeks of hard graft I found myself a sort of amateur expert and felt I could hold my own when the cognitive behaviour therapy people got in touch.

I had no idea that I was barking up the wrong tree.

★

I was sitting at my desk when the phone rang. I have an office in the attic where I do my writing, and after my morning walk I 'commute' upstairs at about eight thirty. I am a disciplined writer, but I like the taut urgency of the deadline as it ratchets a notch nearer each day. Douglas Adams, who wrote *The Hitchhiker's Guide to the Galaxy*, said he loved deadlines — he liked the whooshing noise they made as they flew past. That's not me. I am conscientious. I never deliver late. It is part of my stickler personality.

I had been constructing a paragraph about the Turin Erotic Papyrus, a thousand-year-old illustrated document depicting some Ancient Egyptian men and women having a bit of an orgy. Apart from the drawings of their admirable gymnastics, the orgy scene contains many illustrations of musical instruments and, tellingly, wine vessels. It seemed to me that the way I was using alcohol to relax my stressful inhibitions before and during social occasions — the booze-and-schmooze idea — was not new. The Erotic Papyrus showed that the story of wine, women, and song was as old — older — than the pyramids.

My musing was cut short by the jangling of the phone.

'Hello?!'

'Is that Mr Thomas Cutler?'

Nobody calls me Thomas except my mother.

'Who's calling?' I asked.

'This is Paul Hattman ... From Talk the Talk, the talking therapies service.'

It all came back to me: they had sent me an anonymous-looking letter a couple of days before, saying that I should expect a phone call, and stressing the care they took to protect clients' privacy. It all seemed a bit cloak-and-dagger, and I wasn't sure either, feeling the way I did, that 'client' was the right word. But I decided to be friendly.

'Oh yes,' I said, 'I was expecting your call.'

Paul said that he was an 'assistant trainee psychological wellbe-ing practitioner'. It sounded a bit of a mouthful. Was he qualified in anything, I wondered, and what did he actually do?

The way it worked, Paul explained, was that he would go through a questionnaire with me over the phone and would then pass on my responses to SunBurst. Before long I would be contacted by somebody who would explain how the cognitive behaviour therapy exercises on the website should be done and would then respond online to the 'diary' comments I would be making.

'Okay,' I said, 'Shoot!'

I don't know why I said 'shoot'. Perhaps I thought it made me sound more dynamic than I felt.

Paul asked me several questions, which he was plainly reading off a list. There is a sort of fuzziness to communication when some-body is doing something else while you talk to them. I guessed Paul was keying my answers into some sort of online form. In the end he said he would sum up our discussion in a letter, and rang off.

The next couple of days continued as normal. It was a bitterly cold January and we were getting through the logs at a galloping rate. I was still waking early.

One morning, I looked down into the street from my office window. The pavement was silky with frost and a small icicle hung from the pediment over the door of Captain Henry Roberts' former house, opposite. I imagined the handsome Roberts in his periwig and fancy breeches, meeting my gaze from his window, across the years. He had sailed on the *HMS Discovery*, making maps for Captain Cook, and died in the West Indies in 1796 after getting yellow fever. Like all of us, he had his problems. He was at the mercy of his anguish, his heartache, and the thousand natural shocks that flesh is heir to. Wasn't I making too much of things? Shouldn't I pull myself together?

The sound of the whistling postman snapped me out of it. Amongst the unasked-for catalogues was a letter from Paul 'summarising' our phone conversation. We had agreed, he said, that I 'would benefit from an initial intervention of computerised cognitive behavioural work on SunBurst'. This surprised me.

'We did not agree this,' I replied in a letter. 'Far from agreeing that I would benefit from CBT, I remain open-mindedly sceptical, which I regard as the rational way to approach anything untried, and something which may fail, and which does fail in some cases, though not in others.'

Pedantic as usual. I didn't want to sound contrary, but we were off to a bad start. In any event, I got no reply to my letter. But I did soon get an email from someone called lulu.pickering at SunBurst explaining how their website worked and telling me to do a couple of exercises. Lulu would check in to the site a few days later, and weekly thereafter, guiding me through the online CBT forest.

The SunBurst site was busy and bright, illustrated with potato-print pictograms of men and women. Some of them had brown skin, others had white skin. On the 'What we do' page was a short introduction. This is what it said:

Our user-friendly flexible-access solution-delivery platform comprises a library of interactive empowering programs offering supportive feedback for a diverse range of mental and behavioural health issues. Exploratory and nonlinear, our unique care-path insight and motivational content, including mood charting and interactive journaling, facilitates enhanced engagement and effective service-user retention and completion.

Pardon? Why did I feel I was being done over by a high-pressure salesman?

On the rest of the site there were various sections with headings like, 'Understanding Feelings' and 'What's Your Thinking Style?' Over the next two or three weeks I logged on and went through some of the pages. It was a mixture of Grandma's old-time common sense, fatuous multiple-choice quizzes, and what I will term, for fear of sounding ruder, 'undiluted moonshine'. One inanity, plucked at random, read:

> Word Prisons — Having rules about how you or others 'should' or 'must' behave, and making judgements based on these rules.

I responded like this:

> It's not being in a prison to have rules about how you should behave. It is the guiding principle of every religion, all lawmaking, and all moral philosophy, from the school playground to a G20 summit. I don't need this mumbo jumbo from the Nutty Professor.

In one diary entry, I wrote:

> After looking at the SunBurst site I actually feel worse than I felt beforehand. Surely this can't be the point.

In due course, Lulu replied:

Hi Tom, If you find that your difficulties with the website continue would you prefer to be on the waiting list and not engaging with the online therapy?

I took a deep breath and counted to ten, which I suppose is the plain man's cognitive behaviour therapy from the time before cognitive behaviour therapy. Lulu's suggestion that I stop using SunBurst felt like constructive dismissal to me. Had she waded beyond her depth?

★

I am sometimes accused of being overly critical. Cognitive behaviourists have a name for this so-called 'focus on the negative': they call it the 'mental filter', the idea being that you dismiss or 'filter out' the positive in your life and 'filter in' only the negative. This is said to be bad. But surely alertness to error, weakness, and flimflam can be a useful quality. My fault-spotting has always been one of the handiest tools in my work.

I remember a particular occasion from my early days in the publishing industry when we were preparing to publish a book that was to be manufactured using several elaborate techniques: special acetates, extra colours and varnishes, foils, laminates, and fancy embossing. The designer and I had to go to the print works to proof the job on press, which means viewing the first samples of each printed sheet — every one of which contains numerous pages, half of them upside-down — and adjusting the colours and whatnot before the machines are run up to speed. The print company had put us in a room with a window overlooking the print floor. Here they had made available comfy sofas, coffee, and cakes, and a vast viewing station for inspecting the inky-smelling sheets as they came off the press.

The designer and the print director were bent over a sheet, paying particular attention to registration and ink colour as I floated around, seemingly purposeless, glancing sidelong at the paper with my eyes lidded. Suddenly I noticed something.

'You've lost an arrow on page 76,' I said.

Page 76 contained an elaborate diagram featuring a series of small white arrows amid a riot of text, numbers, and coloured squares. Taking out a lens, my two assistants squinted at the tiny marks on the huge sheet, before lifting their heads and looking at me open-mouthed.

'How in the name of God did you spot that?' said the designer.

'*Upside-down*,' said the printer.

I couldn't say how I'd done it. It had just leapt out at me like a face with a missing eye.

'You're a bit odd,' said the designer, 'but I'm glad you're here.'

Like many writers, I am unsparingly critical not only of myself, but of everything around me. And it is this which I suppose CBT tries to change. I often have to button my lip at somebody's slipshod cooking or a language error in a wedding invitation. But sometimes I speak up. This is a mistake. There is no good to be had from pointing out these things. I have had to learn that people do not want you constantly criticising them and underlining their weaknesses. A woman once told me, 'You spoil *everything*.' Maybe it was right for cognitive behaviour therapy to moderate fault-finding in everyday life.

However, the point of CBT is presumably not to make your clients feel worse than they do already, and I wondered whether therapy with a live human being would be any better than the website — was there really anything in it?

We were into February and I was restless and tense. Lea could tell, but she knew I wouldn't speak about it. I was hardly being fair. Every morning as I examined the bedroom ceiling in the darkness, the knot in my stomach would tighten as I thought of the day to come. It was a struggle to write but I kept my nose to the grindstone.

Weeks passed with no news. By now, spring was on its way and I began to track the progress of the sea kale as it threw out its first shoots from under the barren shingle along the beach.

At the end of March, a letter arrived telling me that I had an appointment with somebody called Odette Pinard, Psychological Therapist in Primary Care (Cognitive Behavioural Therapist). I was asked to come along to the medical centre on 20 April — at the savage time of eight fifteen in the morning — bringing with me the enclosed questionnaire, which I should complete (*underlined*) with a record of my mood over the preceding week. I couldn't help remembering that 20 April was Adolf Hitler's birthday. I hoped it wasn't a bad omen.

I jotted down a remark in my notebook, thinking that I might one day be able to write something about what was happening to me. Every writer cannibalises his own life, and everything is potential material.

Mon, 18 Apr. 2016

I'm going through a slightly mad phase again, but I'm booked in to see some CBT lady on Wednesday. Oh to be boringly normal.

The following recollections of what occurred from then on come in part from the few CBT session sheets which I have kept, and my diary notes.

As requested, that Wednesday, I rolled up at what used to be called the doctors' surgery and is now known as the medical centre and sat down in the waiting room. I was as usual much too early.

About ten minutes before my appointment, a forlorn-looking fellow in a frayed military tie emerged from the end of the passage. His hair was neatly combed but was in need of a wash. He was making an effort to look smart but there was a hole in the elbow of his raincoat and one of his trouser hems was trailing. On the way out he caught my eye and gave me one of the saddest smiles I have ever seen.

I looked over the form I had filled in about my mood during the previous week. Running down the side was a series of questions on depression and anxiety. The depression questions covered things like lack of pleasure in doing things, insomnia, and problems concentrating. The anxiety questions concerned worry, edginess, irritability, and restlessness. I had to tick a box for each question arranged in a series going from 'Not at all' to 'Nearly every day'. I had ticked quite a lot of 'nearly every day's in both sections, with anxiety winning on points.

The sound of a female voice made me look up: 'Thomas Cutler?'

Standing at the end of the corridor was a middle-aged lady, nicely turned out, with a heavy necklace that swung as she moved. I gave her one of my standard two-second 'Pan Am' smiles and stood up.

The 'Pan Am smile' is the name given to the artificial smile said to have been flashed by members of the cabin crew of Pan American Airways as they welcomed passengers aboard. Also known as the 'polite smile' or the 'Botox smile' it involves a perfunctory

CHAPTER 1: FALLING ROCKS

contraction of the muscles that lift the corners of the mouth. A proper smile reflecting genuine emotion is called a Duchenne smile, after the neurologist who identified it as involving not only the mouth but also that vital component, the crow's-feet muscles around the eyes.

I always think I'm smiling a proper Duchenne smile, but people say that when I think I'm smiling I'm actually frowning. I was astonished recently when somebody showed me a series of photographs of myself at a wedding. Everyone around me was smiling beautifully. I looked positively unpleasant.

The lady with the swinging necklace smiled back a cool, expert smile, turned, and walked briskly down the passageway. Clearly I was meant to follow her.

She kept a couple of yards in front of me and I observed her technique as we approached a door at the end, where she stopped, bent forward, and opened it efficiently. She turned and smiled again, holding the door for me. She seemed experienced, which was a bonus, and her practised routine had doubtless become embedded over the years. Her body language was saying, 'I am an accomplished professional who knows her business. I'm a good listener but will not put up with any nonsense.'

'Have a seat,' she said deliberately, letting the door hiss closed on its mechanism.

With a barely detectable accent, she introduced herself as Odette Pinard. She was already calling me 'Tom', but it was unclear whether I had permission to call her Odette or whether I ought to call her anything at all. Maybe it was her Frenchness, maybe her briskness, or maybe all newcomers to CBT feel slightly on the back foot. In the end I settled for calling her nothing at all and kept to this rule until the close of our final meeting.

Odette explained what the plan was, outlining the sessions, of which there would be an initial six. Towards the end we would do a review to see whether we agreed that progress was being made. If it wasn't we would think about my trying something else.

'It's not like psychoanalysis, which can go on for years with no apparent benefit,' said Odette. 'It doesn't suit everyone.'

Was this good sense or a CBT get-out clause for the inevitable failures? I decided to think positive.

Each week, she explained, she would review my mood form and my 'session bridging worksheet' and discuss the progress I'd made, along with any problems I had had during the last seven days.

'CBT is based on the idea that thoughts, feelings, and actions are interconnected,' said Odette, 'and that negative thoughts and feelings can feed on themselves. We try to tackle problems in practical ways; we won't be going back over your past very much.'

This approach sounded more congenial than dredging up a load of childhood family relationships. A practical attack was more my cup of tea. While I have always found the conjectures of Sigmund Freud suggestive, I am sceptical about the usefulness of psychoanalysis. On one occasion when Freud was at a psychoanalytic conference with one of his famous cigars in his mouth he was asked if he was not aware of its phallic implications. 'Sometimes,' he retorted, 'a cigar is just a cigar,' which sounds like the usual Freudian escape ticket, of which there always seems to be one to hand.

Having written this cigar quote down, I did what I always do and checked it out to see if it was authentic. What I found was that Alan Elms, a sometime psychology professor, discovered years ago that there is no record of the remark before 1950, more than a decade after Freud's death. He concluded, disappointingly, that it was too good to be true.

Checking and correcting are typical of me. If there's a wonky picture I must straighten it. If a door is open to the wrong angle (according to my own rules) it troubles me and I have to get up and adjust it. This used to drive Lea nuts, but she now grudgingly indulges me. If I am getting petrol I am obliged, by little squeezes of the pump trigger, to get the petrol meter and the price to display precise whole numbers with no decimals, and it is almost impossible to get both to do so simultaneously. All this is pretty exhausting.

Odette said I would have a fifty-minute session once a week for six weeks. We would work together to tease out the thoughts, physical feelings, and actions connected to any problems I had had, and try to adjust my thinking and behaviour if she felt they were unrealistic or unhelpful. I would then go away and try to practise these techniques, and report back.

While I listened, I scanned the room. It was a windowless purpose-built space, with a desk against one wall. There were two hard chairs, separated by the corner of the desk upon which sat a large computer. The lighting was chilly and there were no pictures. At the junction of wall and floor, the vertical plaster met the concave skirting, which curved into the smooth floor covering, with a line of white mastic visible at the intersection. It was as if the allowance of sharp corners in such a room represented the very antithesis of cleanliness and health.

'So how did you get on with SunBurst?' asked Odette.

I told her the gory details of my unhappiness with the website and its various idiocies. I went on about this in some detail and stopped only when I found myself shaking with anger.

'No human being should have to put up with that kind of thing!' I barked.

I was aware of Odette looking at me. Was my reaction in

proportion? Probably not. She was writing something down.

'So how have you been feeling?' she asked.

My outburst hung in the air like gun smoke.

'I've lost all my mirth,' I replied.

I'm not sure Odette got the reference.

'Like Hamlet,' I added.

She had a look at my mood sheet, making notes on the computer as she did so. I'd ticked 'anger' and 'irritability', 'restlessness', 'memory and concentration problems', and 'difficulty making decisions'. I hadn't ticked 'Thoughts of harming yourself'.

'Let me explain how CBT works,' she said.

I bent over the table to get a better view as she sketched out a diagram.

'The first thing is the trigger. It's: "Trigger, Thoughts, Feelings, Behaviours."'

She drew arrows connecting the four headings in a sort of circle.

'What I'm going to ask you to do next time it happens is to write down the *trigger* situation that's causing your negative feeling. For example, someone might have been critical of you, so you write that down, okay? Then you write down what *thoughts* this triggers. It might be, "I'm not good enough", or something like that. Next, write down the physical *feelings* this has caused in you, you know, like annoyance, or resentment, or whatever. Then finally you put down your actions, your *behaviour* — what you actually did. It could be something like, "I made a defensive excuse."'

She tapped the pencil on the table to show she had finished.

'You're looking confused.'

'Not confused,' I said. 'It's just that that's not the way it is. There's no trigger. I wake up niggled and I stay niggled. I've always got this knot in my stomach.'

Odette rubbed the back of her neck.

'How much alcohol do you drink?' she asked.

I explained that I medicated my anxiety with it and that it worked. She became brisker. Unless I could cut my drinking right back for the next six weeks, she wasn't convinced that CBT would help me.

'It compromises the therapy,' she said.

We then had a long discussion in which I queried the whole notion of alcohol units. It was a pointless piddly argument and we were both becoming irritated. I decided that the situation needed rescuing.

'All right,' I said, 'I'll do my best to cut down the alcohol and I'll fill in the paperwork as you suggest.'

'Oh good,' she said. 'Well, time's up. In fact, we've gone slightly over.'

Odette stood and handed me the session bridging sheet to fill in for next time. She held the door open. 'See you same time next week.'

She gave me a smile. It looked more Pan Am than Duchenne. As I went down the stairs I cleaned my hands with the alcohol gel I always carry. I felt, as usual, that I'd got off on the wrong foot. At home I made a note in my diary:

Quite hard work this morning owing mainly to my refusal to leave my brain at the door. I was reminded of Bertrand Russell, who, when his brother was trying to teach him some mathematics, asked why he should believe the axioms of Euclid. His brother replied, 'Well, if you don't we can't continue.' This is how I felt today, having to accept the dubious axioms of CBT or we couldn't continue. Trouble is, my argumentative insistence that some evidence of their truth should be given seemed to annoy the therapist. Came home feeling angry, but I don't know why. Everyone says I always seem so calm but there's this constantly suppressed rage.

Having promised to moderate my drinking for the six weeks of the CBT I decided to cut it out altogether. I am a black-and-white thinker. With me, it's all or nothing. I stayed off the drink entirely for the next two months.

During the first week of CBT, I kept a lookout on my thoughts, feelings, and actions, and scribbled down a few notes for the following session. It rained a lot that week and I had to take an umbrella to my next meeting with Odette Pinard.

Weds, 27 Apr. 2016, session 2

Wet and windy today. Going up the stairs to the waiting room I had to pass that jazz mural in banana yellow and fluorescent green. All those zigzags, sharp edges, and screaming colours. Hospitals and doctors' surgeries are full of this rubbish. It's enough to give you an epileptic fit.

'Any feelings about last week's session?' asked Odette.

'Yes,' I said, 'this room. If I were designing a consulting room I would never use cold blue lighting like this. It's an elementary mistake. This place ought to be warm and inviting but it looks like somewhere cadavers are dissected. There are no plants, no rugs, no softness. And that mastic down there is not smooth. Whoever put it on didn't take enough care. How can people be expected to relax in an environment like this?'

Odette was looking at me quizzically and writing something down.

'So what is it especially about these lights?' she asked.

'Well, first the colour temperature is too low — they're cold. Second, they're fluorescent. They're making my head spin. It's like the supermarket. I find those places impossible: fluorescent lights, all those people, all that noise, and the turmoil of all those shelves, all those labels, all those smells, all that bloody advertising. It makes me scream.'

I was breathing hard. I received another puzzled look.

'Your depression and anxiety scores are about the same as before,' said Odette languidly, going over the sheet. 'How has your week been? You said last time that you were finding social situations *"taxing"*.'

'Still very difficult,' I said. 'We're going out to dinner in three weeks with a couple of friends and I'm already starting to get tense. One person I can manage. Two is more difficult. Three is absolutely exhausting. I could just say no and let them get on with it, but it's not fair on my wife. Anyway, I want to fit in, so I go along with things. I have learnt over the years — trained myself — to imitate what other people do in social situations, because I don't seem to know how. I'm always pretending to like it, to be someone else. It's exhausting.'

Odette was writing again. Was it me or was there the flicker of a smile on her lips? She looked up.

'You know, Tom, people who report similar behaviours are not only exhausted by the constant performance you mention, it's what causes much of their depression.'

She gave me a booklet: 'Low mood — your self-help guide'. The title was printed in three separate type styles and three different colours. It was hard to take. At the foot was a cartoon blob-man in a hat, a jaunty question mark above his head, printed in yet another typeface. I took it away with me. It was still raining.

As the sessions progressed I seemed to be treading water. I read the sheets I was given: 'Following your heart', 'Activating yourself'. There were picky arguments. I complained about the cup dispenser for the water cooler in the waiting room which was so badly designed that it dispensed three or five cups at a time. At the end of May I reported intense irritation at people wearing sunglasses, so that I could not tell whether I was being looked at.

My nightmares were continuing, and I kept waking in the early hours. Lea was being patient. Odette advised me to implement a 'sleep hygiene' process by sticking to a rigid routine. Bed at eleven thirty, no reading. Up at five thirty. The same every night. Miraculously, it seemed to work. I wasn't waking early so often. As for everything else, it remained static.

In session five we were due to review progress, but a few days beforehand I got a message changing the time of the appointment. I hate changes to my routine. Hate them. There was nothing for it, however, so I made a note to turn up an hour later than usual.

When I arrived, the waiting room was empty. There was a newspaper on the table: 'HACKER SUSPECT HAS NERD SYNDROME SAYS DOC.'

Odette appeared at the end of the passageway and we did the follow-her-up-to-the-door routine. We went in and I sat down.

'Well, Tom, how do you think things are going?'

I sucked my teeth.

'I don't think it's working,' I said.

'It's not, is it!'

Odette looked at me long and hard, with her head on one side. Her initial chill had changed somehow. She seemed to have warmed to me.

'You know what,' she said, 'I've been thinking about your first session, when you told me in great detail about your objections to the SunBurst website. When I listened to you then I wondered, "Have we got something else going on here?"'

I noticed a spider scaling the wall. It was struggling to make progress, the smoothness of the paint providing little purchase. While I was silently egging it on it fell back, being stopped in midair by a thread of invisible silk. In a twinkling it was off again, climbing towards its goal.

'How do you mean, "something else"?' I said.

'Think of these points. You say you find social situations "taxing": you have taught yourself how to fit in but you feel as if you are always pretending — people find you aloof; you get a sensory overload in busy shopping centres; and you have a special interest in road signs — in one session you talked at some length about the London Tube Map —'

'It's a diagram, really, not a map,' I said.

'There! You're a *details* man and a *rules* man: definitions, commas, errors, corrections — *didactic interruptions*. Now taken together, along with some other peculiarities, I think all this might be pointing to something.'

I stiffened. Was I being primed for something nasty?

'I'm wondering, Tom,' said Odette, 'whether you might be on the autism spectrum. At the high-functioning end. Asperger's syndrome.'

'Balls!' I exclaimed, without thinking.

I knew that people with Asperger's syndrome could be bluntly spoken but anyone might have responded like this.

'No,' I insisted, 'I've worked with Asperger's people and I've read about it. I'm not like that. I'm not a geek. Nothing against geeks, I like them, but I've got a sense of irony, I get jokes. That's not me.' I felt as if I'd been struck in the face by a leather belt.

Odette gave me an encouraging smile. She seemed completely relaxed.

'You told me you have a degree in Fine Art. Now think about it. You could have been interested in Classical sculpture, or abstract expressionism, or the Dadaists. But no, your special interest is the design of British road signs. This is a very uncommon and particular interest. Transport signs are systematic, and the autistic mind loves systems.'

'But I'm coming at it from a design point of view. *Aesthetics*,' I said weakly.

I felt as if I was sinking — up to my waist in sand. Her remarks had bothered me. I had never thought about it before, but now I stood back for a moment this enthusiasm of mine did sound like a typically autistic subject.

The spider had reached a light switch and to continue had to decide whether to go left or right.

Odette drew a line. 'The Asperger's people you've met might be down here on the spectrum. Further end. And you might be up here at the more subtle, abler end. A bit harder to spot. I think this really might explain your longstanding anguish.'

I made my just-smelt-a-cesspit face.

'Have a think about it, Tom. Go away and read about it and come back and tell me what you think next time. That's due to be our final session.'

My head was a blur. Surely this was nonsense. I took a left out of the medical centre. I always turn left if there is a choice. It is a rule I rigidly stick to. Coming out of an underpass I will always take the left exit even if I know I will have to cross the road outside to get to where I want to be. Like many of my other rules I keep this one to myself but I dislike varying it. Was this a bit odd? Was it a bit autistic? I made my way home as if I'd just been told that I might have a chronic but interesting tropical disease.

There was a lot to think about. First the panic attack, then the anxiety diagnosis, and now this. Was Odette making wild guesses or did she have something? Over the past few weeks I had become less sceptical of some of the things she said. After all, I was sleeping better.

I have an interest in Sherlock Holmes; I've read all sixty stories in the canon many times, and I thought then of one of my favourite Holmes quotations: 'It is an old maxim of mine that when you have excluded the impossible, whatever remains, however improbable, must be the truth.' If I could eliminate the impossible perhaps this Asperger's syndrome idea might prove to be the truth. If I looked at my difficulties from this new point of view might it explain a few things? Could it explain everything?

I felt I had been given a treasure map, but there were holes in it. I needed to fill them in. I would start by finding out all I could about autism and Asperger's syndrome, and we would go from there. It could be an adventure.

I put my key in the lock. There would be a lot to report back on next week. But first I must tell Lea.

I picked up the phone.

Chapter 2:
Signals not in use

Asperger's syndrome
(also **Asperger syndrome**)

NOUN

A developmental disorder related to autism and characterized by awkwardness in social interaction, pedantry in speech, and preoccupation with very narrow interests.

Origin: Named after Hans Asperger (1906–80), the Austrian psychiatrist who described the condition in 1944.

On a bare strip of coastal plain hard up against the chalk skirt of the South Downs National Park nestles the sleepy seaside neighbourhood of Lancing.

At low tide, walkers in quilted windcheaters exercise their dogs along the wet sand, swinging in their fists small plastic bags of something. Here and there, like a new tooth in an old mouth, a piece of contemporary architecture glistens heroically between the beach huts, rotting groynes, and guano-splotched nursing homes. But most famous of the town's landmarks is the gigantic neo-Gothic chapel of Lancing College.

I rise from my train seat as the chapel slides past us on its hilltop, away to the right, buttoning my jacket against the late spring breeze. I am on my way to an appointment with one of the country's most notable experts on Asperger's syndrome. I'm hoping she will be able to tell me whether I've got it or whether something else is going on. If I can discover, as I hope, a reason for my years of oddball confusion and give the thing a name, perhaps the mists will clear.

I had been itching for a formal assessment from a specialist ever since Odette Pinard's canny guess that I might be on the autistic spectrum. I use the word 'assessment' rather than 'diagnosis' because it sounds less medical: the difference between having something identified that is not an illness but which is causing you problems, and being pronounced diseased, disordered, or dysfunctional.

I had been reading as much as I could about Asperger's syndrome, which is a mysterious and complicated condition. I remember sitting down on the first day and flipping through a basic primer. After a bit, I started to laugh. It was the laughter of recognition. This was a stark reflection of the essential me: the solitary nature; the aloofness, the dislike of change, the special interests, my inability to chat, my pedantry, my sensory peculiarities, my suffering in company.

When I had mentioned to Odette at our last session that I was planning to ask my doctor to refer me to an expert she had shaken her head. 'Attempting to get a positive identification that way,' she said, 'will be like trying to squeeze champagne out of a walnut. And you'll be waiting about two years for an appointment.' Two years was certainly no good for me. My need to understand what had been making me feel so out of sync for so long was pressing. I wanted to get on with it.

Lea had been pretty non-committal about the suggestion that I might have Asperger's and my decision to look for an expert opinion, but I was on tenterhooks. At last, after years of bemusement, I could see an answer emerging like the shadow of a lifeboat through the fog. Things were coming into focus and all the strange feelings and faux pas over the years were beginning to make sense. Still, I could hardly expect my wife to deck the place in bunting and throw a party.

We are drawing into the station. This train is a new one, with a foul colour-scheme and automatic toilet-doors that open of their own accord while people are in there. As we pull alongside the platform I look over my shoulder for my hat. As I always must.

The ticket barrier is one of a sort I have seen before, and I have very little difficulty with it: a minor victory this, because I often get in a muddle with automatic barriers, card payment gadgets, and ticket machines. Anything more than the simplest un-smart phone is beyond me.

On a ticket machine I recently counted nineteen separate places that I had to pay attention to before I could select, pay for, and collect my ticket. I cannot 'block out' irrelevant information and find myself concentrating on all of it, including the details of the manufacturer stamped on the metal, the corrosion on the screws, the texture of the brushed steel, and the temperature and feel of the various bits as I touch them. Together with the generally poor ergonomic design, the maddening instructions, and the incomprehensible navigation, all this jangling overstimulation causes my anxiety to build to such a degree that I cannot take in any more information. I cease to function properly and become enraged, often with a queue breathing down my neck. Onlookers generally see this as an infantile overreaction. Outbursts of this kind, which are common among autistic people, can be so intense that they are known as 'meltdowns', a nickname borrowed from the dictionary of nuclear disasters.

All the same, despite the abolition of helpful bus conductors and railway guards, never mind all the train lateness and cancellation, the unexpected timetable changes, and the uncomfortable closeness of other passengers, public transport it is still easier for me than driving. I got rid of the car years ago having become exhausted by the plethora of information I had to process while behind the wheel: other vehicles, traffic signs, commercial signs, unexpected road works, changing lanes, changing gears, changing weather, changing road surfaces, tarmac smells, speed bumps, speed limits, tight seatbelts, changing down without the brake, nattering passengers, bleeping seatbelt warnings, sudden diversions, ticking indicators, plastic smells, petrol smells, petrol stations, boys on bikes, air conditioning, honking and hooting, satnav, mirror-signal-manoeuvre, traffic cones, screen wash, people giving you the finger, people disobeying the rules — which are there for a reason — people waving you through, pedestrians, potholes, one-way streets, windscreen wipers, *plus* my pressing need to turn left, which was creating some interesting but unnecessarily long journeys. 'You need to relax a bit,' Lea had told me for the umpteenth time. 'Why can't you be normal for once in your life?'

As I come out of the station, I pause for a moment to watch a departing train. Like traction engines and pumping stations, trains are a frequent preoccupation for autistics. I look over at the dilapidated frontage of an abandoned Art Deco cinema, built in 1940: the year Alfred Hitchcock made *Rebecca*, his film featuring the indescribably creepy housekeeper, Mrs Danvers. L U X O R it says in flaking letters. The cinema is to be converted into 'luxury apartments', or what used to be called small flats.

The gates of the level crossing are closed so I climb the steps of the old railway bridge. Halfway over I notice four steel plates welded to the green superstructure, each studded with twelve rivets. These rivets appear to me as a pattern, like the dots on a domino. I run my hand over the bumps as I pass. They are cold but not unfriendly. I like bridges. They are built to systematic physical rules that make sense. They don't confuse me. They are solitary, as I am. They keep still.

Under my arm is a folder containing the pages of notes I have put together while reading up on autism, of which Asperger's syndrome seems to be a subset as mysterious as autism itself. It is a fascinating subject, but too often larded with long words and unhelpful jargon. The American stuff I have seen is especially rich in this sort of thing.

Take the following terms plucked at random from various books, magazines, and websites: *assistive and augmentative communications* (AAC), *broader autistic phenotype*, *weak central coherence*, *applied behavioural analysis* (ABA), *assistive technology*, *pervasive developmental disorder — not otherwise specified* (PDD — NOS). None of these names tells you what it means, as *earache*, *walking stick*, and *yellow fever* tell you what they mean. 'Assistive technology' is just *helpful equipment*;

43

why dress it up in such gaudy clothes? And how anybody could accept without laughing a diagnosis of something named 'pervasive developmental disorder — not otherwise specified' I don't know.

If I wanted to get my head around this subject I would have to translate this loopy slang into a self-explanatory vocabulary that looked like English, instead of something off the home page of the Intercontinental Confederation for the Promulgation of Obscurantist Acronymicality and Latinate Sesquipedalianism (ICPOALS).

One of my first troubles was not, though, the daft initialisms and fancy words but the simple lack of a noun for a person with Asperger's syndrome. If you have asthma you can be, 'an asthmatic' or, adjectivally, just 'asthmatic', but this isn't possible for a person with Asperger's syndrome. People have had a stab at creating a suitable word, with 'Aspie' being the front runner. But this sounds coquettish to me. It would have been possible to keep referring to 'a person/people with Asperger's syndrome', though that's quite a mouthful, and one which might annoy those who dislike what's known as 'person-first' language.

Person-first language is a cart-before-the-horse linguistic device that results in such cumbersome formations as 'a person with sight loss' and 'a person with Asperger's syndrome'. Person-first language insists that diabetics must no longer be called 'diabetics', they must be 'people with diabetes'; the bald are not to be called 'the bald' but 'men with hair loss'.

The online encyclopaedia Wikipedia says that person-first language is 'a disability etiquette designed to avoid perceived and subconscious dehumanisation when discussing people with a health issue or disabilities'. I'm pretty sure that 'a health issue' is what we used to call 'an illness', 'injury', or 'disease', but what 'perceived and subconscious dehumanisation' is (or are) I can only guess. Are you really less than fully human if you are blind, diabetic, or bald?

In his 1999 essay 'Why I dislike "person-first" language', Jim Sinclair, who is autistic, makes the important point that autism is not something you have, like an injury or disease, so much as the fundamental essence of who you are. So, 'a person *with* autism' does not even make sense.

There is a never-to-be-settled debate grumbling away about all of this, a debate often carried on, rather incongruously, by people who are not themselves autistic. The autistic, bald, and blind presumably have bigger fish to fry. Anyway, if a woman with hearing loss wants to call herself deaf that's fine by me. It is shorter, more vigorous, and less fuzzy. Nobody should be ashamed to be called autistic, nor *to be* autistic, any more than they should be ashamed to be asthmatic. I suppose that if one of my friends were a necrophiliac he might not want to be described by that term in the pub, but calling him 'a person with necrophilia' isn't going to help. I use the term 'autistic' without demur.

As for the lack of a noun for people with Asperger's syndrome my answer has been to create my own: *Asperger* (singular), *Aspergers* (plural). For example: 'There is no such thing as a typical Asperger' and 'Aspergers find social situations confusing'.

★

It was while I was exploring the Aladdin's cave of Asperger's syndrome that I came across the details of Sarah Hendrickx, who was giving a lecture to the UK's National Autistic Society. Sarah is an experienced diagnostician and consultant, but she is more than that: together with her academic qualifications she brings to the job a unique sort of understanding because she has Asperger's syndrome herself. That she worked just along the railway line from me was an unexpected bonus, and I had dropped her a note to make an appointment.

Taking a slip of paper from my pocket, I refer to the directions on it: *Take left, follow street till reach big pub with green roof. From there follow nose to SH's office.*

After a few minutes walking I spot the street I'm looking for. I've been told to pass through a tall gate, taking care on the other side not to approach the door on the right but to ring the bell beside the door straight ahead of me. These instructions suit me well. They have plenty of specific detail and no ambiguity.

I glance at my watch. Just as I intended, I am forty minutes early. I feel extremely uncomfortable arriving late for anything: a meeting with a friend; a train; a dinner; a film showing. I cannot go into a film if the adverts have started. Because of my twitchiness I often find myself arriving an hour early for an appointment, having caught the train before the one I was supposed to get. But today these forty extra minutes will prevent my being late and also allow me to plan and manage my arrival.

Having identified the office, I smartly pass it by, crossing over the road towards a small park, where I sit down on a bench beside a pole-mounted receptacle intended for dogs' excrement.

A magpie lands on a nearby branch. The magpie is a highly intelligent bird: the only non-mammal which can recognise itself in a mirror. Although I have a rational distaste for superstitious mumbo jumbo, I also have an irrational suspicion of lone magpies, for, according to the nursery rhyme, one magpie is for sorrow. I feel my heart quicken. Is this bird a bad omen? Superstitions of this sort, I've read, are common in people with Asperger's syndrome.

CHAPTER 2: SIGNALS NOT IN USE

I scan the park, as is my routine, in the hope of finding a second magpie. I spot one lurking among the copper beeches. Like a placebo pill, this second bird relaxes my anxiety. Two for joy: that's a relief.

How can a logical, rational, and clear-headed sceptic like me be alarmed by such utter tosh? For years I have deliberately walked under ladders and opened umbrellas indoors to show myself what I think of this kind of superstitious rubbish, but a single magpie still makes me jump. It is one of my secret horrors.

I look at my watch and have to look at it again to see what the time is. My meeting is in sixteen minutes. I leave the park and nose around the area for ten minutes or so. A man in a fluorescent vest is getting out of a council vehicle. From the top, a long, cantilevered arm swings a concertinaed pipe out towards a drain, like a great elephant's trunk preparing to suck up a drink. As a child the noise of these drain suckers used to terrify me.

I go into a corner shop, where I buy something small. I come out and walk among the clumps of suburban housing. The street furniture is painted in a variety of murky greens. In the distance the crown of a wooded hill rises above the bungalows. Many of the lawns and flower beds around here have been replaced by tessellated grids of cement bricks on which sit gigantic cars of various colours. One front yard has subsided in the corner, causing an eerie disintegration of the pattern of interlocking tessellations. This bothers me.

I pass a house with a *Mon-Repos*-type sign next to the front door. *The Dogs Danglies* it says. I note the missing apostrophe. The sign's substrate is a thinnish piece of brushed steel with the characters printed on top in a curly brown script intended to resemble brush-drawn letters. But it's been done by machine. In a high window, I see a child's mobile rotating slowly. I watch it closely for a minute. It is only later that I discover the autistic penchant for spinning objects.

I check my watch. My appointment is in six minutes so I retrace my steps, adjusting my stride to arrive back at Sarah Hendrickx's gate precisely twenty-five seconds before my appointed time. I ring the bell with eleven seconds to spare.

The door is opened by a smiling woman who looks a few years younger than me. If she's got Asperger's syndrome you'd never guess it. Of course, you can't tell just by looking. We go through the greeting nonsense and she ushers me up the stairs and sees me into her office. Do I want coffee? Tea? I should make myself at home.

I look around the comfortable room and spot several books with titles like *Asperger Syndrome and Alcohol: drinking to cope?*, *Asperger Syndrome & Employment*, and *NeuroTribes: the legacy of autism and how to think smarter about people who think differently*. I take this one down. It is a big fat book by a person with the name Steve Silberman. Its cover is decorated with a grid of twenty-five small rectangles in two different blues. Lost among the rectangles is the book's long subtitle, being four lines of condensed capital letters printed in three different colours, one for some reason upside-down. The author's name is at the head and, below it in a fourth colour, the name Oliver Sacks: the man who wrote the foreword. The cover is further confused by a badge showing that the book has won some sort of prize. I find honours and prizes distasteful, though when I later come to read the book's five hundred and ninety-two pages I discover it to be a work of art. All the same, the overactive design is not something I imagine anybody with Asperger's syndrome wanting to look at.

Sarah comes in with the tea and I plonk myself down on the sofa. There is a small circular table for my use, on it a glass of water. I notice that many tiny bubbles have settled on the wall of the glass. This tells me that it has been sitting here for some while. Clearly

Sarah prepared for my visit in very good time, possibly even before I started my own mental preparations in the park, forty-odd minutes ago.

'You found me all right then.'

I recognise that this statement of the obvious is intended to start the ball rolling. I daresay Sarah has learnt to do this, just as I have learnt to respond with a trite confirmation.

'Yes,' I say.

There is plainly no exchange of information going on here. Nobody is learning anything they didn't know before, but I have come to understand over the years that a conversation of this sort is not about information exchange. It has instead an important social function, like the discussion of the weather by two old men at a bus stop. People call it 'chitchat', or, if you start a conversation with it, 'breaking the ice'. I have absolutely no natural small talk of this sort, and though I have learned to imitate what other people do on these occasions, and can sometimes give a plausible impression of being almost as capable of idle prattle as anyone else, I feel a fraud while doing it. It's a formula. I'm pretending to be someone I'm not again.

'I got here forty minutes early to check things out,' I add, sensing that 'Yes' was possibly not enough to qualify as full-blooded chitchat.

'Did you?' says Sarah Hendrickx, frowning curiously, 'That's not something most people would do.'

'Isn't it?' I say.

Sarah gets down to business and the conversation develops over the next couple of hours, with me talking about my strange life and some of my awkward experiences, while she nods and listens. This is followed by questions that she reads off a form, and which I answer while she writes things on a sheet of paper.

'Do you like silliness?'

'Actually, I do,' I say. 'I love silliness of all kinds. Why do you ask?'

'Oh, it's a fairly common trait among people with Asperger's.'

'And normal people without Asperger's,' I remark donnishly.

'Yes, and not everybody *with* Asperger's. Some take the world extremely seriously. But for many there's an oblivious disregard for pointless social conventions, a childlike curiosity, and an enjoyment of "inappropriate" activities like running up the down-escalator, for example, or trying on all the hats in the shop, that kind of thing.'

This makes me think. When I worked in the office of an accountancy firm near St Paul's Cathedral the partners used to tell me that they liked their people to have a sense of humour. But if I ever put the stapler on my head, or made a silly face or witty observation, which I sometimes used to do, I would find them looking at me as if their finger had gone through the toilet paper. Humour — what they saw as idle facetiousness — was not thought 'proper', no matter what they pretended.

There is a loud roaring from outside. It could be the elephant machine emptying the drains. Sarah shuffles her papers, searching for something, and excuses herself for a moment.

A hard sun is striking the furnishings, causing ranks of diagonal stripes to creep across the carpet, here climbing a chair leg, there sweeping slowly across a windowsill. I look down at my notes and see something I've underlined: *Is Asperger's syndrome a subset of autism?* Then, underlined twice to show me it is a cardinal question: *What exactly is autism?* This is followed by some scribbled 'case histories' from the distant past, the first of which concerns a child whose strange behaviour was recorded more than two hundred years ago.

★

In 1794, or thereabouts, a French doctor named Jean-Marc-Gaspard Itard (1775–1838) told the extraordinary story of a handsome child of about twelve who was noticed living naked in the woods near Saint-Sernin-sur-Rance, a village in southern France. He seemed to have been abandoned.

The so-called 'Wild Boy of Aveyron' was later caught by some hunters and brought to a nearby town, where an official wrote that there was 'something extraordinary in his behaviour, which makes him seem close to the state of wild animals'. Itard called the boy Victor.

Victor did not speak, could not understand tones of voice, and seemed incapable of learning more than the rudiments. He had unusual food preferences, and would rock himself repeatedly back and forth. Persistent food fads are common among autistics, who also find rocking, hand flapping, spinning, and leg jiggling to be soothing. In modern parlance, these calming actions are known, somewhat contrarily, as 'self stimulating' behaviours, or 'stimming'.

For five years, Dr Itard tried to help Victor to talk and to become social, but till the end of his days he remained aloof, almost totally unable to communicate or make attachments. He died of pneumonia in 1828, probably in his early forties.

At more than two hundred years old, this account of what looks very much like autism is one of the earliest direct records that we know about. There is certainly no reason to doubt that the condition stretches far back into human prehistory, but the trouble is that trying to identify autism from historical writings is a game of pinning the tail on the donkey, so one has to be very careful. All that can really be said about Itard's observations is that they are intriguing.

The real breakthrough description of autism, in the way it has now come to be understood, was made in America, in 1943, at the height of the Second World War. Leo Kanner, an Austrian-born psychiatrist, who was working at Johns Hopkins University School of Medicine in Baltimore, wrote a remarkable paper: 'Autistic Disturbances of Affective Contact', 'affective' here meaning, *having to do with the emotions*.

Kanner had identified the 'autistic' condition in eight boys and three girls. One of them, a boy named Donald, came to his attention in a letter sent by the boy's father. In thirty-three pages of obsessive detail he explained how his son was happiest when alone, living within himself and oblivious to everything around him. He would shake his head repeatedly from side to side and obsessively spin himself or his toys in circles. When his routine was disturbed, temper tantrums would result.

Meeting Donald, Kanner observed that he referred to himself in the third person, was explosive and abnormal in his use of language, and repeated words and phrases that had been said to him. He realised that Donald, and all the children he was describing, shared features of a unique condition previously unidentified, or at least, so far, unnamed. They had almost no desire for social contact and were just not on the same wavelength as other children. The fundamental problem, he explained, was:

> The children's *inability to relate themselves* in the ordinary
> way to people and situations from the beginning of life
> … There is from the outset an *extreme autistic aloneness*
> that, whenever possible, disregards, ignores, shuts out
> anything that comes to the child from the outside …
> He has a good *relation to objects*; he is interested in them,
> can play with them happily for hours …

The effect of Leo Kanner's lucid descriptions was immediate: the pattern of behaviour he had observed was recognised at once by others.

Among his assumptions, however, were some that turned out to be false. He believed that autism affected only children, but had he watched them over time he would have seen that they grew into autistic adults, and that their autism remained with them for life.

He also made little of his children's cognitive impairments, instead singling out their ability to do puzzles, and their adroit handling of inanimate things.

We now know that something like half of all autistic people have a learning disability, and many have epilepsy or another problem from a range of recognised physical conditions. Some need full-time care, perhaps from a parent, or in a specialist institution. Autism pioneer Uta Frith has noted, however, that, despite their frequent intellectual challenges, autistic children are often, 'remote, beautiful, and mysterious', like those in John Wyndham's novel, *The Midwich Cuckoos*.

But, the most damaging of Kanner's assertions was the false idea that autism was a result of bad parenting, especially by emotionally cold 'refrigerator' mothers. Over succeeding decades, this disastrous error was to occasion enormous harm to autistic children and their grief-stricken parents. Today we know that the emotionally frigid mother doctrine is unequivocally false. Autism is not the result of incompetent or negligent mothering any more than freckles are.

In the 1940s, the long shadow of Sigmund Freud still darkened the consulting rooms of Europe's white-coated mind doctors, and German-speaking psychiatrists fleeing the European war rhapsodically exported Freud's curious fancies to the United States, where they took off, spawning a psychoanalysis fad that continues to this day. Gradually, however, good scientists dropped fruitless Freudian mind-reading in favour of investigations into what seemed to be going on mechanically inside the autistic brain.

Autistic brains show some intriguing features. They are physically different: the connections are different, the structure is different, various areas behave differently and look different; and sometimes they are bigger and weigh more. Post mortem autistic brains typically have many more neurones than the common brain. The brains of non-autistic people who have congenital differences in their corpus callosum — the bundle of two hundred million nerve cells connecting the two halves of the brain — have been linked with the following problems: trouble grasping non-literal language, difficulty understanding other people, clumsiness, seizures, and poor face recognition; all traits common in autism. These same brain differences have also been tied to such things as an enhanced knack for language and languages.

The senses of autistic people are unusual. They may be uncommonly attuned, or 'hypersensitive' to sounds, smells, tastes, touch, and visual stimuli.

Most people remember overall impressions, but autistics concentrate on detail, sometimes being unable to see the wood for the trees. They often spot details and connections that others miss, and they are quick to notice when something has changed. They tend to favour facts, patterns, and repetition, and will insist on doing things in their own way: they might always eat the same foods, wear the same clothes, or walk the same routes, and they can become highly distressed when expected, for example, to eat a different breakfast or sit in a different chair.

Autism is present from the early years and the signs can be seen in babies, who may not gurgle or smile, might not point or make eye contact, and who, when they cry, may not want to be comforted. Sometimes, however, the condition seems to emerge later, after more typical early development. The child might appear to be progressing as expected until all at once his or her behaviour mysteriously begins to regress.

The handicaps of more severely affected autistics are occasionally counterbalanced by extraordinary spikes of scientific, musical, or artistic talent and creative imagination. This marked difference is known as 'uneven skill development', or what Uta Frith has described as 'islets of ability' in a sea of disability.

The idea of the so-called 'autistic savant' struggling to communicate and take care of himself, yet able to play the piano and guitar at the same time, or draw from memory a detail-packed panorama of London, has been featured so often in films and on television that a notion has grown up that many autistics have gifts of this kind. But this is untrue. Autistic savants are exceedingly few and far between.

In 1944, a year after Leo Kanner's influential paper, another Austrian paediatrician, Hans Asperger (1906–1980), independently used the word 'autistic' in a work of his own. It is debatable whether Kanner and Asperger happened upon the same coinage by mere serendipity. The word 'autism' was little more than thirty years old at the time, having been minted in 1910 by a Swiss psychiatrist called Eugene Bleuler, who derived it from the Greek *autos*, meaning 'self', and used it to describe the self-absorption of schizophrenics. Being already in clinical use it might well have seemed just the job for describing the inwardness of the children that Kanner and Asperger both wrote about.

Hans Asperger, who worked in Vienna, had studied hundreds of different children and singled out four boys between the ages of six and eleven. The behaviour of these children bore some similarities to that of Kanner's eight boys and three girls.

Both groups had social problems and difficulty with relationships, but, unlike Kanner's autistic children in America, Asperger's boys had no learning difficulties. They were bright sparks, intensely absorbed in their own areas of interest. Asperger called them 'little professors' because they could talk in detail about particular subjects in which they took great interest.

But, though they had large vocabularies, these children were aloof, their conversational style being 'transmit only', and they did not seem to grasp the unwritten rules that govern two-way social behaviour. Being brainy is not enough. For success in life you must be able to get on with other people, and the children Asperger had identified had trouble with this.

People with Asperger's syndrome find it difficult to establish friendships despite making gauche attempts to do so. They may have no *savoir-faire*, and chatting can be a mystery to them. Their social approaches are often made in such a naive, forlornly inappropriate way that communication founders, and this is not a trivial matter; even in adulthood they can find themselves victims of teasing and occasionally physical attack. It is hardly a surprise that a large number of Aspergers suffer clinical depression, as well as anxiety.

Aspergers are also more likely to be dyspraxic, which is a nicer word for 'clumsy', and might struggle to tell left from right. Sometimes they will have a lazy eye or bowel problems. Their gestures can be few or peculiar, and they might move in a quirky way, for example, by walking on their toes with a loping gait. There is frequently a lack or unusualness of facial expression and eye contact. They may speak in a strange unmusical monotone and use language in an odd way. They might interrupt others, and can be pedantic, stilted, or inappropriately formal. They also frequently speak too loudly, and have to be told to shush in restaurants and museums. Despite their odd speech, Aspergers are frequently good with the formalities of language, often establishing large vocabularies and sophisticated syntax, though — paradoxically — they are also more likely than the general population to have dyslexia.

They can be highly accomplished and creative artists, scientists, actors, musicians, and writers, but their abilities often conceal problems with organisation and planning. Dylan Taylor, a handsome young autistic man, describes himself as 'never a school person', but at the time of writing he holds the record for the highest cumulative score in the history of *Countdown*, a British television word-game. His knowledge of the darkest corners of the *Oxford English Dictionary* is astonishing. From a random selection of nine letters he managed to produce *septarium*, which is the word for a certain sedimentary nodule, and in another round *elasipod*, a deep-water sea cucumber. Though impressive, this is not a vocabulary suitable for striking up new friendships at a cocktail party or smoothing the way in a job interview.

Unlike diabetes, there is no blood test for Asperger's syndrome. The question 'Has X got Asperger's?' is like the question 'Is X in love?' Forensic science will not help you. Deciding whether someone has got Asperger's depends to a degree on detective work, long experience, and a certain amount of circumstantial evidence. But, as Sherlock Holmes remarks, 'Circumstantial evidence is a very tricky thing. It may seem to point very straight to one thing, but if you shift your own point of view a little, you may find it pointing in an equally uncompromising manner to something entirely different.'

When I was young, the circumstantial evidence of my

'oversensitive' personality and unusual behaviour did seem to some people to point in another direction. My offhandedness and pernickety grammar, my insistence on wearing the same old-fashioned clothes till they were mere rags, and my anxious solitariness, led my mother and some of my teachers to describe me in the then fashionable vocabulary of psychoanalysis. Mercifully I was never accused of having a 'castration complex' or of being an 'anal-sadist'; the term that kept cropping up was 'sensitive'.

Anybody with Asperger's will also have a personality independent of the autism, but the two will be tangled together. Much later, when I was grimly struggling to find out why I'd always felt so bewildered, I took a well-known personality test. The results described me as a rare type known informally and rather grandly as 'the Mastermind'. Masterminds are said to be concrete thinkers, introspective, logical, rational, and clear-headed. Though open-minded, they are strong-willed and decisive. They aim for the highest quality in what they do and insist on the best from others. They can be effective leaders but tend to step into the breach unenthusiastically. Their single-minded concentration on their own ideas can cause them to ignore people's wishes and feelings. It certainly sounded like me.

I had spotted Isaac Newton's name on a list of famous people of this Mastermind personality type, though he was identified elsewhere as having many of the classic characteristics of Asperger's syndrome. It was all very mysterious. There seemed to be as many questions as answers.

Some of the other traits of Asperger's syndrome are listed in the superb 'Autism Toolbox' designed for schools, and first published in 2009 by the Scottish government:

- Difficulty in grasping people's meaning and intentions
- Perceptual differences
- Concrete thinking focused on facts, physical objects, and the here and now
- Organisational difficulties, such as trouble getting started
- Indifference to incentives or praise
- Distractibility
- Poor awareness of relative importance
- A literal understanding of language

Whether these oddities have been naturally selected or are just by-products of something else, is not clear. In the world of autism research, little is clear and nothing is static for long.

Like classic autism, Asperger's syndrome is a complex and deeply puzzling lifelong neurodevelopmental condition that affects the way the brain processes information and experiences the world. It is seen as part of the wider autism spectrum, sometimes cropping up in families where classic autism is also present. But the question is how the learning difficulties and below average IQ that often go along with classic autism can be part of the same picture as the high-functioning, articulate, and self-aware presentation that one sees in Asperger's.

Is it the genes? There are many leads but few answers, and this situation is frustrating for researchers. If both classic autism and Asperger's are due to the same genetic liability, why do some people have the full picture and others only the so-called 'milder' problems?

Asperger's syndrome is, indeed, occasionally referred to as 'mild autism', but for many whose lives are a daily social or sensory obstacle course, or who have been made profoundly unhappy by the condition, 'mild' is not the right word.

Despite their undoubted intellectual capabilities, many Aspergers struggle to find work. In 2018, the National Autistic Society reported that in the UK only sixteen per cent of autistic adults were in full time employment. It is at the interview stage, where social poise is tested as much as skill and experience, that Aspergers often fail. The three magic questions in an interviewer's mind are: 1) Can you do the job? 2) Will you do the job? and 3) Will you fit in? It is the last question that usually does for the shortlisted Asperger. Even if he does get the job he can find collaboration hard. Expecting such a person to obey the incomprehensible plexus of social rules, which have been written by non-autistic people and which prescribe 'proper' behaviour, is just forcing an day upon an owl.

★

The term 'Asperger's syndrome' only gained widespread popularity after it was used, in 1981, by English psychiatrist and autism pioneer Lorna Wing (1928–2014), who was also the mother of a classically autistic daughter and had already spent two decades as one of the founder members of Britain's National Autistic Society. She was to become an inspiring worldwide influence on the evolution of new ideas about autism.

Wing's hugely influential paper 'Asperger's syndrome: a clinical account' introduced the idea of an identifiably different presentation of autism, challenging Leo Kanner's long accepted model of a rare condition with a narrow range of traits. She and her colleague Dr Judith Gould proposed instead the highly influential insight that the features of autism are spread across a spectrum, not just of severity but also of variety, and that every autistic person appears somewhere on this 'spectrum'. At its most subtle end, says Wing, 'the spectrum shades imperceptibly into eccentric normality'. Steve Silberman suggests that this is the most 'subversive' idea embedded in the concept.

The core deficit across this spectrum is the social one; it is a lack of 'social imagination' — the ability to use the imagination in social contexts. But despite the blurring along the line, there is a difference between the epileptic autistic with a low IQ, who does not speak, cannot dress himself, and who will climb out of high windows if left to his own devices, and the research scientist who is obsessed by soap bubbles, wears strange hats, and finds shopping centres intolerable.

A recent idea is that the autism spectrum should be looked at as an example of 'neurodiversity'. The concept is that not all brains are wired the same, that everybody in the general population has his or her own strengths and weaknesses, that brains develop in different ways, and that people's differences should be much more readily accepted at school, at work, and in everyday life.

Neurological differences in the general population have not evolved out, and many people with Asperger's continue to attract mates and breed successfully. So the traits of autism may be just another example of general diversity in the environment.

Human beings resemble other animals in this respect. Look at a pack of dogs, each with its own skills and foibles. One will be an aggressive leader, another a cheerful rounder-upper, another, more alert and anxious than the rest, will wake from a doze quicker and scent danger before the others. It is the same with people. One will be a great organiser, another a good morale booster, a third will be rather aloof, a bad diplomat, the unseen watcher, not joining in around the camp fire but sitting alone and alert against a tree, waiting. Perhaps it will be this person, the one with the autistic traits, who smells the forest fire sooner, who hears first the warning snap as the creeping enemy breaks a twig underfoot. Perhaps.

★

Having given Asperger's syndrome a name and brought it into the autism fold, Lorna Wing didn't have to wait long for the authorities to start raising objections. The Asperger's syndrome jack was hardly out of the box before people were trying to force it back in again, and by 2015 the World Health Organisation was calling it 'a disorder of uncertain nosological validity'. The American Psychiatric Association took the condition out of the 2013 edition of its bible, the *Diagnostic and Statistical Manual of Mental Disorders*, nineteen years after having first put it in, introducing a new term, 'autism spectrum disorder', which now covered everything. Wing, who died in 2014, had few complaints about this. She believed that the drawing together of everything under one 'autism spectrum disorder' umbrella would lead to better understanding.

But many single-minded people with Asperger's syndrome turned up their noses at its replacement in the DSM, instead clasping 'Asperger's' to their bosom, careless of whether it was recognised by the American Psychiatric Association or not. They did this on the grounds, possibly, that it was already theirs and, unlike 'nosological validity', did not sound like a pompous sock of mud.

Some, no doubt, also saw 'disorder' as rather a rude word to use. Once upon a time, homosexuality was described as a disorder, but the medical and psychiatric establishments finally thought better of it. One of the most influential authorities on autism and Asperger's syndrome is Simon Baron-Cohen, Professor of Developmental Psychopathology at Cambridge University and Director of the

University's Autism Research Centre (ARC). Baron-Cohen has pointed out that 'disorder' is such a prevalent word these days that people who sometimes lose their temper are now being diagnosed with 'intermittent explosive disorder'. On the other hand, maybe there is sense in calling a spade a spade. Anyone who thinks that Asperger's is not a disorder might like to have a conversation with someone who is living with it. In any case, the Autism Research Centre has made the decision to use the more neutral term 'condition'.

Though many people do find Asperger's a great burden in their lives, some also find its intellectual, creative, and focus-concentrating blessings a compensation, preferring to see it as a 'difference'. There are always arguments about terminology, and some people complain that a formal identification of Asperger's syndrome does little more than hang an unhelpful label around people's throats. Many who meet the diagnostic criteria for Asperger's say they get on fine in their everyday lives without a formal diagnosis. As Tennyson put it, 'That which we are, we are', and some are perfectly happy to be that which they are, without having a tag clipped to their ear. As usual, Lorna Wing put her finger on it: 'The diagnostic labels don't mean a damned thing — just use them to get the person the services they need.'

One of the most intriguing features of Asperger's syndrome is the drive to dig deep into uncommonly intense and narrow subjects of interest. These peculiar fixations or obsessions are known to professionals as 'special interests', though many have adopted other less clinical words, such as 'enthusiasm' or 'passion'. The 'obsessive' drive to look deeply into particular subjects is a trait that blends into the ordinary enthusiasm for certain hobbies which is common in many people, most especially boys and men. Perhaps the archetypal autistic enthusiasm is train spotting: the solitary figure in his anorak, doggedly logging and systemising, as all around him people go about their business.

Aspergers tend to be notably independent thinkers, and the array of 'special interests' is astonishing in its variety. Such enthusiasms are often for mechanical, quirky, or systemisable subjects — it might be tornados, baseball or cricket scores, ice-skating, steam trains, antique mousetraps, moths, etymology, dams, the stock market, dinosaurs, astronomy, television comedy shows, bus timetables, US presidents, deep fat fryers, *Star Trek*, or, as in my case, British road signs. The list is full of crazy variety. Sometimes it will be a fascination for collecting a particular category of objects, such as fossils, automata, or thimbles. Some interests are so specialised that few can match the knowledge of the Asperger's expert. I met one chap who knows more about lifts than perhaps anyone in the world.

Occasionally an Asperger's enthusiasm can be for another person. When this person is Abraham Lincoln nobody minds, but new friends on the receiving end of such oppressive attention can find it unnerving.

One of my own special interests is Sherlock Holmes. In her 1989 book, *Autism: explaining the enigma*, Uta Frith says that Sherlock Holmes has something that looks very much like Asperger's syndrome. He is, she says, not merely eccentric: his absent-mindedness in relation to other people and his single-mindedness in relation to special ideas are classically autistic traits. She mentions his detachment and his circumscribed interests, giving as an example his monograph, 'Upon the Distinction between the Ashes of the Various Tobaccos', in which he enumerates one hundred and forty ashes, from cigar, cigarette, and pipe tobaccos.

Holmes has a number of these special interests. He is an accomplished violinist and an obsessive expert in practical chemistry, as well as an authority on newspaper typography, secret writing, and all the different kinds of London mud. Dr Watson is put off by the foul chemical smells with which his flatmate fills their Baker Street home, but takes particular exception to his most antisocial interest, indoor marksmanship:

> I have always held that pistol practice should be distinctly an open-air pastime; and when Holmes, in one of his queer humours, would sit in an armchair with his hair-trigger and a hundred Boxer cartridges and proceed to adorn the opposite wall with a patriotic V. R. done in bullet-pocks, I felt strongly that neither the atmosphere nor the appearance of our room was improved by it.

Since childhood, I have felt an affinity to Sherlock Holmes, his solitariness, his specialised enthusiasms, and his strange quirks and habits, such as smoking the dottles of the previous day's pipes in his first pipe of the day, his musical ability, his seriousness, his silliness, his emotional chill, his disdain for mere convention and the supernatural, the huge gaps in his general knowledge, his fastidious cleanliness, his weird sense of humour, and his firing revolvers indoors for fun. Apart from the gun business, he reminds me of me.

In fact, the Sherlock Holmes stories are generously sprinkled with Asperger types. In *The Hound of the Baskervilles*, for instance, we have Dr Mortimer, an untidy, absent-minded physician and amateur archaeologist who scribbles notes on his cuff and has a special interest in skull anatomy. Then there is Stapleton, a butterfly-mad naturalist who obsessively classifies his catches, pinning them to cards. And Mr Frankland, a pedantic eccentric with that key Asperger trait, a rigid and quirky personal sense of justice, whose preoccupation with the technicalities of the law causes him to fight cases for the mere pleasure of fighting.

But it is Sherlock Holmes' solitary brother Mycroft who takes the Asperger biscuit. He has a mania for detail, an unbendingly constrained routine, a phenomenal memory for facts, and a horror of company so great that he is joint founder of a club that forbids any member to speak to any other. Holmes describes him to Dr Watson:

> He has the tidiest and most orderly brain, with the greatest capacity for storing facts, of any man living … his specialism is omniscience … Mycroft has his rails and he runs on them. His Pall Mall lodgings, the Diogenes Club, Whitehall — that is his cycle.

In Sherlock and Mycroft Holmes, Arthur Conan Doyle has given us an illuminating portrait of two Asperger types, each with his own unique palette of idiosyncrasies.

Some people know only the austere Asperger's stereotype — the strangely dressed geeky man who won't shut up about his special interest, except at parties where he closes down entirely, or the badly behaved boy who will not look you in the eye and has infantile tantrums if he can't get his way. But there is no such thing as a typical Asperger: people are affected in different ways and to varying degrees. Every person with Asperger's syndrome is in some way different from every other person with it, each with his or her own assortment of traits. In fact, people with this syndrome are more different from each other than are typical people in the general population. It can look so unlikely that the self-assured, piano-playing, beautifully turned-out toastmaster who remembers the name of every guest at the Mansion House dinner can truly share the same condition as the cheerful chatterbox with fluorescent hair who is an expert on bees, or the absent-minded, scruffy-bearded, apprehensive, pedantic engineering student who eats nothing but egg sandwiches. But thrust unexpectedly into an informal group of chatting people they will reveal themselves to be fellow travellers, all at sea, their dependable moorings cut.

Asperger's learn in a different way and seem to deal with information to do with emotions and social situations by using a process quite at odds with that of the typical population. It is as if their user's manual is printed in Thracian, so they have to learn the social game intellectually and by imitation. It can be a struggle for them to make it through the day, simply because of their problems getting to grips with the mysteries of other people. Often they feel that others do not understand them. Even when they form firm relationships there is frequently a strange remoteness at their core. Dr Watson tells us that Sherlock Holmes 'loathed every form of society with his whole Bohemian soul [and] remained in our lodgings in Baker Street, buried among his old books ...'

At parties, which are a special kind of torture for them, Aspergers may stand alone in their odd outfit or attach themselves, limpet-like, to a friendly-looking person. Often they will dodge social situations altogether and do a bit of computer programming or catalogue their music downloads at home instead. They will be used to the complaint, 'Why do you never let your hair down?'

They are also said to lack a sense of humour, but this is quite untrue. Many are highly amusing people: some are great raconteurs, others are wits, while still others make their living as stand-up comedians. Their idea of what is funny can, all the same, strike people as bizarre, or objectionable.

The film director Alfred Hitchcock was renowned for his

peculiar taste in humour, practical jokes, and racy stories. Though he was generally known as Mr Hitchcock he reputedly urged some people to address him by his foreshortened nickname. 'Call me Hitch,' he would say, 'Hold the cock.'

I have always admired and enjoyed Hitchcock's films, and I had recently read that he showed signs of Asperger's syndrome. When I went to my books about the great director and re-watched some of his television interviews I began to smile at the number of suggestively autistic qualities in the man.

The signs were there from childhood. By the age of eight he had ridden the entire length of every bus line in London, and if that doesn't tip you off about his autistic tendencies then you have no soul. By fifteen he had got a job as a draftsman in an engineering firm. Engineering is a trade that crops up repeatedly in the families of Aspergers. It is the application of mathematical and scientific rules to the design, analysis, and operation of structures, machines, or systems; a system being a combination of things that are working together as parts of an interconnecting network. Systems and systemising, not necessarily mechanical, are a speciality of the autistic mind. Professor Simon Baron-Cohen gives filmmaking as a good example of a system.

Hitchcock was well known to the television-watching public for his show, *Alfred Hitchcock Presents*, and to cinemagoers for his walk-on appearances in his own films. In interviews he was often oddly unsmiling. His gaze could be peculiarly oblique, and when answering queries he frequently looked away. Some people found him alarmingly aloof and off-putting. His deportment was passive, accompanied by a quiet, peculiarly monotonous speech style in which he delivered concrete, sometimes pedantic, answers to interviewers' questions.

He lived by unbending rules, a classic Asperger trait, whether in filmmaking, manners, or dining — another of his enthusiasms. As part of his rigidity, Hitchcock insisted on reading the London *Times* in Hollywood. He always dressed in a dark suit, white shirt, and black tie, his wardrobe containing many suits of identical funereal style. When shooting *The Man Who Knew Too Much* under the intense heat of the Moroccan sun his only concession to the sweltering atmosphere was to discard his jacket. I understand this sort of behaviour entirely. People often say to me, 'Aren't you hot in that outfit?!' as I sit awkwardly on the beach in my three-piece corduroy suit.

Hitch was impeccably polite, if cool, and insisted on the same decorum from others. Lateness he would not put up with. He loathed conflict, and on the few occasions when an actor flared up, he fled the set. 'I am shy, you know,' he told Fletcher Markle in 1964. 'I'm not very gregarious. I don't mix with a lot of people …' Actress Linden Travers explained: 'He wasn't the sort of person that everybody could go up and chat to … He was quite … remote and self-contained.' Nonetheless, his longtime colleague Norman Lloyd remarked that for a man with 'so definite a point of view and so definite a personality' he was 'most respectful of other points of view'. This openness to hearing conflicting opinions is typical.

Though he could be intermittently playful, Alfred Hitchcock was didactically earnest about his overriding special interest — filmmaking. To him, the pre-production engineering of the film was the interesting bit. Shooting he found tiresome.

He propounded a system of rules for constructing a story, which he had acquired from his English screenwriter Eliot Stannard. These rules created constant anticipation and suspense that kept the audience wanting to know 'what happens next?' He would spend months building the suspense architecture of his stories, and when he had finished, would make a shot-by-shot map of the film on storyboards, the ultimate visual planning system.

Hitch took some of his stories from popular novels. But though he admitted to reading a great deal he said that he never read fiction for pleasure. The tendency of those with Asperger's syndrome to prefer non-fiction to fiction has been much discussed. One idea is that they lack understanding of social relationships, so that novels do not generally attract them, preferring instead the more 'lawful' world of facts and figures. Hitchcock certainly *wrote* a lot of fiction, but that is a different thing entirely. Indeed, some critics have complained that in his films the interpersonal relationships are abnormally contrived and peculiar.

Hitchcock had a highly anxious dread of authority, and he funnelled this into his films. Norman Lloyd remarked that, 'The anxiety is what has made him one of the major artists of the twentieth century.' Hitch explained that he enjoyed playing the audience like a musical instrument. 'I don't care about content at all,' he said. 'The film can be about anything you like so long as I'm making that audience react in a certain way to whatever I put on the screen.' For a person who finds social situations hard to control or even understand, this method of regulating other people in a predictable way, through a system of cinematic rules, is greatly pleasing, rather as a conjuring trick is to a magician.

It is not unusual for Aspergers, who may seem aloof and indifferent, to form unusually strong attachments to certain preferred people: they might be girlfriends or boyfriends, or new friends. These powerful attachments are sometimes one-way, and it is not surprising that this can unsettle people. The problem in Hitchcock's case was that he became attached in this highly focused way to beautiful icy blondes, in the Grace Kelly mould, over whom he became uncomfortably proprietorial. He oversaw the design of their wardrobes and exerted control over their private lives. Tippi Hedren, who later accused Hitchcock of making unwanted advances, broke off her personal and working relationship with him, at great professional cost, though others, including Grace Kelly, managed to keep him as a friend.

Hitchcock's directness — often perceived no doubt as bluntness — might be what made him so good with children, who are often the same way themselves. Actress Veronica Cartwright, who sixteen years later was to do a lot of screaming and whimpering in *Alien* (1979), remembered Hitchcock interviewing her in his office for the part of the young girl Cathy Brenner in his film *The Birds* (1963). He decided, in typical Asperger style, to talk to the twelve-year-old about one of his enthusiasms — wine. He told her about the best wine distributor in Bristol, the town of her birth, and recommended particularly good vintages. 'These things of course I've applied in later years,' Cartwright remembered, 'but at the time ... I thought, what an odd conversation.'

When Hitch was asked what he might have liked to have done if he hadn't made films, he replied, 'I think it might have been amusing to have been a criminal lawyer.' This is an ideal job for a person with Asperger's syndrome. It has a firm, unambiguous, systemised structure of unchanging predictability, sameness, rules — not to say laws — and non-social, non-reciprocal communication, with more than a dash of performance thrown in — something in which Hitchcock admitted to taking a 'hammy' pleasure.

★

Like law, mathematics is a structured system, and the Autism Research Centre found more autism diagnoses in maths students than they did in those studying the humanities. In the other sciences they discovered more autistic traits, though not more autism.

Most Aspergers have a mathematical ability that falls in the usual range, somewhere along the typical bell curve. A few, though, are uncommonly gifted, appearing well outside the average, at the extreme high-performance end, while others find the subject unusually difficult.

I myself find numbers tricky and mathematics very difficult, though this is balanced, I suppose, by my knack for words. It is an example, I guess, of 'uneven skill development', the tendency for autistics to have deep troughs and high peaks in their abilities.

The variations in severity and the great variety of ways in which Asperger's characteristics are intermingled can make it hard to identify the condition in, say, a member of your family. You cannot tell that someone has Asperger's by looking at him or her, and there is a tendency for people to reject the idea that someone who is bright and articulate, if a bit strange, can be suffering significant problems every day. For this reason, Britain's National Autistic Society calls Asperger's syndrome a 'hidden disability'.

Until quite recently, Asperger's had simply gone unidentified and un-understood; now, more and more people are being spotted, if sometimes rather late in life. In the past they would commonly have been regarded as mere nutcases, misfits, or eccentrics, no doubt having wondered for years what was going on, and why they felt so lost.

Take Matthew Robinson, second Baron Rokeby (1713–1800), a wealthy English eccentric of the old school.

An impossibly shy man, Robinson led the life of a hermit, and had probably always been odd. Though polite, he seemed to have what one contemporary described as 'too much of the phlegm of the philosopher for him to appear amiable'. Many men shunned him for his strangeness, and women were said to find him uncanny. He disliked company and his rare visitors found themselves obliged to sit for hours, shifting from one aching buttock to the other, as he recited long poems of excruciating dullness, unaware of his guests' deep boredom.

As a young man, Robinson travelled abroad to see the sights, and it was upon his return from the German spa town of Aachen that he became an obsessive fan of baths, bathing, and water in general, drinking pint after pint of the stuff all day for years.

When he inherited the family estate in 1746, he arranged for a hut to be built on the nearby beach at Hythe and made lonely trips to the ocean every day to swim, heedless of the English weather. He had drinking taps put into the ground at regular points along the way, and when he spent too long in the water, as he often did, his manservant would drag him unconscious onto dry land.

Having converted his greenhouse into a bath, which was supplied by a spring, he would lie in it for hours, his unfashionably long silver beard spreading over the surface like pondweed. All his meals were taken in this bath, his unchanging diet consisting of beef tea, venison, and water.

Lord Rokeby held strong idiosyncratic convictions, supporting freedom of religion, thought, behaviour, trade, and animals, and though he kept human visitors at bay, he allowed horses, bulls, cows, sheep, goats, and dogs to wander freely over his estate, and liked to march about before sunrise, dressed up in a farmer's outfit.

He lived to be eighty-seven, spending much of his life alone, drinking water in the bath. He died in 1800, having never married.

Good old English eccentricity is one thing, but Rokeby's

insistence on sameness, his monomania, his peculiar tastes in food, his strong and unusual personal convictions, his favouring animals over people, and his solitariness and social oddity, look very much like attributes of autism. He was, of course, never given an Asperger's diagnosis because there was no such thing to be had. These days, fortunately, Aspergers are increasingly getting support — if they need and want it.

The English aristocracy appears to have a rich historic seam of autistic crackpots running through it. This is not because the nobility are especially prone to Asperger's syndrome, but because their money and connections mean that people want to write about them.

Scientist–aristocrat Henry Cavendish (1731–1810) was another of these rum ducks, who in 1766 had discovered hydrogen. Vastly wealthy, Cavendish at one time had more money in the Bank of England than anyone else, and kept houses in central London as well as one in the country, at Clapham Common. It was here, in typically inventive style, that he decided to weigh the Earth in his garden shed using a piece of kit consisting of two pairs of lead balls and a fine wire. He published his phenomenally accurate result in 1798.

But Cavendish was known as much for his oddity as for his scientific accomplishments. A character of habit and routine, he walked the same walk every day, like clockwork, dressed in a strangely outmoded suit. He was a profoundly shy man, who deplored society, had no close friends, and spoke in an odd squeaky voice only to men he knew. He was said to have built an extra staircase onto his home to avoid the discomfort of meeting his housekeeper.

In a 2001 article in the journal *Neurology*, neurologist–author Oliver Sacks (1933–2015) referred to Henry Cavendish's 'virtual incomprehension of social behaviours and human relationships' and proposed that he had had Asperger's syndrome.

Sacks himself was an interesting case. A busy neurologist who kept obsessive notebooks in and out of the office, he still made time to write books on the subject of the brain, including *Awakenings* (1973) and *The Man Who Mistook His Wife for a Hat* (1985), as well as works on autism, which fascinated him. In his 2015 autobiography, *On the Move*, Sacks referred to his 'self-absorption', 'solitude', and 'implicit selfishness'. 'It has sometimes seemed to me,' he said, 'that I have lived at a certain distance from life.' He believed that his profound diffidence, which he called 'a disease' and a lifelong impediment to his personal interactions, stemmed from a condition from which he suffered, known as 'face blindness' or 'prosopagnosia' from the Greek *prosopon*, 'face', and *agnosia*, 'ignorance'. Face blindness is more common in Aspergers than in the general population and is associated with the abnormalities in a part of the brain known as the fusiform gyrus, which has also been implicated in dyslexia.

I have a mild form of face blindness myself, and it can get me into trouble. I remember once staying at a friend's house and, in my usual awkward way, introducing myself to another guest. 'Yes, Tom,' she responded, 'we've met. Several times. Like yesterday at dinner.' This kind of thing is always happening to me.

Though not very connected to people, Oliver Sacks was attached to his collection of metal ore and stones. In a highly pregnant remark, he said about his collection, 'I want company, even if it's inorganic.' Late in life he revealed that he had been identified as having 'social phobia or Asperger's syndrome'. Though he believed that this diagnosis 'overstated' it, he grudgingly admitted to being 'an honorary Asperger'. His strange demeanour and odd way of speaking do seem to suggest Asperger's syndrome. However, he felt that some of the truly extraordinary Aspergers he had interviewed for his books were beings of a different sort. For some people, a diagnosis helps; for others, like Oliver Sacks, it doesn't, and there is no point hanging the label on him just for decoration. This is a key point, for unless someone's autistic characteristics are having a damaging effect on their life, which they certainly can have, a diagnosis may be of no use or interest to them. Aspergers differ from one another so markedly that one will look upon his diagnosis as the key that finally opens the gates of understanding and solace, while another will see the label as about as much use as a visa for a country he has no wish to visit. But whatever they feel, they will probably feel it strongly, as in Aspergers the emotion and purpose dials are turned up very high.

Pinning the Asperger's badge to any number of eccentric dead scientists and artists has become the latest seductive parlour game, but you have to watch out because to a man with a hammer everything looks like a nail. In 2003 mathematician Ioan James and Simon Baron-Cohen suggested that Einstein and Newton both showed classic autistic signs, though in lectures Baron-Cohen was duly cautious, admitting that biographies of the dead are a 'fragmented source of evidence'. All the same, maybe Douglas Adams had a point when he observed: 'If it looks like a duck, and quacks like a duck, we have at least to consider the possibility that we have a small aquatic bird of the family Anatidae on our hands.'

In historical cases, there are certainly shared and suggestive signs that point to Asperger's. Typically, the subject is an intellectually bright man, but odd, alone, and averse to human contact. He may be preoccupied with sameness and routine, with his own idiosyncratic ideas and peculiar enthusiasms — sometimes useful, sometimes ludicrous — which he pursues relentlessly. Fashion is of no concern to him. He has a tendency to wear unusual clothes, not merely unfashionable but often from a previous age: an old-style suit maybe or something amounting to fancy-dress.

Some of these men, and as we are increasingly discovering, women, are notably crisp and fastidious; others are remarkably scruffy and disorganised. Often they are inconsistent. Dr Watson describes his flatmate:

> An anomaly which often struck me in the character of my friend Sherlock Holmes was that, although in his methods of thought he was the neatest and most methodical of mankind, and although also he affected a certain quiet primness of dress, he was nonetheless in his personal habits one of the most untidy men that ever drove a fellow-lodger to distraction.

Once upon a time, people such as Cavendish and the water-loving Rokeby were frowned upon; today, we understand more about the context of it all. People like this may seem very strange or they might appear to be fairly typical, if quirky, Joe and Jane Bloggses, charmingly preoccupied with the taxonomy of Namibian birds or mapping the heavens. Judy Rivkin, Executive Vice President of the US Asperger Syndrome Coalition, told the *New York Times*, 'Many Asperger's people seem gifted and normal, and maybe they are in some regards. But that doesn't mean that they don't have to face profound problems.' Most Aspergers long to fit in, to have friends, to be accepted by others, they just don't have the social wherewithal to make it happen.

★

When I was studying Fine Art at university, bohemian parties were a frequent affair. Very much wanting to fit into this world, I would force myself to go, taking on board copious amounts of Dutch courage in advance. But, as others danced or snogged, I usually ended up alone, looking through bookshelves or sitting detached in my rather formal clothes, staring into my glass. Everyone else seemed to have been given the stage directions in advance.

If I gathered the nerve to approach a group and introduce myself, I would manage the whole thing awkwardly and be met with blank stares and furrowed brows. My struggle to carry on a conversation while containing and concealing my fright could make me appear offensively offhand or aggressive. I always seemed to say the wrong thing and people found me brusque, abrupt, or stupefyingly rude, and I would find myself subtly, or forthrightly, repulsed. Thinking back, I suppose I did not seem bohemian so much as unnervingly strange. But when they objected to my presence, it always came as a complete surprise to me. At one party I said something so badly wrong that the young hostess burst into tears. 'Get him out of my house!' she cried, and within seconds two of her rugby-playing friends had deposited me on the doorstep, coat in hand. I was obliged to walk three miles in the rain, back to my digs.

The other thing that often happened was that I would be spotted by some lonely bore, who would gravitate towards me and occupy me for eons on his pet subject: the proper way to coil electrical cables, *Star Trek*, or, on one particularly dire occasion, the serial numbers of drain covers. This drain fan, who was a BBC engineer with a beard, insisted on taking me outside to show me a particularly fine sewer lid. As a man alone at a party, these characters seemed to recognise in me a kindred soul, and would cling to me like garlic skin to a wet finger.

In 1985, a British study looked into the idea that the social problems of autistics are down to the special difficulties they have in understanding the beliefs and wishes of other people. Professor Uta Frith, assisted by Simon Baron-Cohen and Alan Leslie, published an article, 'Does the autistic child have a "theory of mind"?'; that is to say, does he or she understand that other people have minds? Frith and her team concluded that there is, in autistic children, something they called 'mind blindness'. Grasping what others think, rather than what is happening in the physical world, is vital, they said, for complex social activity, cooperation, and learning from one another. A lack of this ability is a handicap. According to Frith, reputation management and political spin are possible only because of 'mentalising' — the ability to put oneself into somebody else's shoes. This word overlaps with the term 'empathising', which Simon Baron-Cohen was to explore more deeply in later years.

People with an impaired theory of mind are said to have a different way of looking inside themselves. Unsurprisingly, they take longer to process social information because they need to analyse situations by using their intelligence rather than picking things up with an intuitive 'sixth sense', as others do. Naturally enough, socialising tends to exhaust them.

Some of the attributes that flow from an impaired understanding that other people have their own mind are the inclination to be breathtakingly honest and the tendency to do and say things which others find rude, disrespectful, critical, or harsh, with the associated lack of understanding that certain subjects are likely to cause embarrassment.

As a child, I was taught that, if offered some cake, I was to survey the plate and take the smallest piece. If there wasn't enough to go around, I was to decline. When visiting Germany as a schoolboy

I noticed that if the Germans wanted cake they said so. If there was a bigger bit, they took it. If it ran out, it ran out. This seemed a better, more straightforward way of going about things, but I often came a cropper and had to learn not to reply to a question such as 'Does this dress look okay on me?' without mulling over the likely consequences of a straight answer. I have realised that an unvarnished expression of opinion is not the right response to such questions, which are intended to invoke approbation. I have to stop myself saying to a woman friend, 'Have you put on weight?', just as a child might ask loudly, 'Why is that man so fat?' Once, when an acquaintance told me he had just had cancer diagnosed, I asked him, 'Will it kill you?' He took offence, but to me it seemed a perfectly sensible question to ask.

Along with forthright straightforwardness there is a tendency for Aspergers to 'overshare'. This ungainly term refers to their impulse to say too much, to give too much personal information. This is especially noticeable in formal situations. 'Sorry I'm late for the meeting but I had to go up to the toilets on the third floor and my fly got caught open' is the kind of thing that makes colleagues wince. Being socially naive, the Asperger might not pick up on the frowns and sidelong glances that tell others in the group that a social error is being made. In most cultures, the penalties for making a social error are severe, and people can find themselves suddenly repulsed, abandoned, or fired.

Importantly, those with an impaired theory of mind can also have great difficulty in reading the messages in another person's eyes. In 1997, the Autism Research Centre created the 'Reading the Mind in the Eyes' test, in which subjects were shown tightly cropped, black-and-white 'letterbox' photographs of the eye-region of a series of human faces and asked to select, from a short list for each picture, a word to describe the emotion in the eyes.

Women in the general population did slightly better than men, and typical people did significantly better than people with Asperger's syndrome. The test showed that normal adults could recognise mental states from the smallest cues, just the subtle expressions around the eyes, and that this ability, to a greater or lesser degree, eluded Aspergers.

A particularly distressing difficulty for brothers, sisters, girl-friends, boyfriends, wives, husbands, and friends is the reduced or odd communication of love and affection that is at the core of many Aspergers. They might express affection very briefly or at low intensity, and often seem puzzlingly cool. Sons or daughters may reject embraces from mothers and fathers, brothers and sisters. Aspergers can be as emotional as anyone else but they must be allowed to show it in their own way. If a greater display of love or affection than they can manage is heaped upon them or demanded of them they may become confused or overwhelmed and go into 'shutdown', a word used to describe the impenetrable withdrawal of autistics into themselves.

★

I once saw a motivational quote in a café. 'Be yourself,' it said, 'everyone else is already taken.' But for an Asperger, being yourself can so often lead to misconception and rebuff, so it is little wonder that many high-functioning autistics find themselves trying to conceal their condition.

In 2017, Laura Hull and colleagues published a study on the website of the Autism Research Centre called 'Putting on My Best Normal: social camouflaging in adults with autism spectrum conditions'. The study looked at almost a hundred adults with a diagnosis of an autism spectrum condition, including Asperger's, who had tried to hide or 'camouflage' their autistic traits in social situations.

The report showed that camouflaging was a common behaviour for people on the autism spectrum and that practice in the required techniques resulted in many being able to pass themselves off as 'perfect counterfeit bills'.

The aim of the camouflaging behaviour was to mask and compensate for autistic traits, and to seem more 'normal'. One subject said that her autistic lack of non-verbal signals was read as hostility, arrogance, or indifference, and there was an almost universal desire among subjects to fit in, and to make connections with others. Although the objectives of camouflaging were often met, the intense concentration and self-control were described as mentally, physically, and emotionally draining, like studying for an exam or interpreting a foreign language. All this I recognise. In social situations I often feel like the man walking downstairs who starts paying attention to his feet. Suddenly losing his instinctive ability, he can no longer control them properly and has to think how to walk.

Strenuous effort and constant self-monitoring are needed during social occasions, and unlike the easy cocktail-party 'impression management' that 'normals' seem to take in their stride, Aspergers reported that the obligation to maintain a constant active camouflage was extremely challenging to their identities.

Subjects of the study often believed that, while successful in the short run, their efforts to 'hide in plain sight' resulted in the manufacture of a facsimile personality, with their 'real' self permanently hidden behind a false front. 'Sometimes,' said one, 'I feel as though

I've lost track of who I really am, and that my actual self is floating somewhere above me like a balloon.'

People masked their conditions in different ways. Chatting was a fearful prospect for most, so they prepared in advance. Some made it a rule to monitor and increase eye contact. Asking more questions was seen as the best deflection and camouflage. One subject described her process: 'I usually ... think up stories and how whole conversations might go before I have them, so I have responses practised, as well as potential things to say if the conversation dries up.'

This rehearsal provided reassuringly structured 'scripts' to fall back on. The problem was, of course, that people sometimes found themselves falling back on a bag of spanners because, despite constant self-monitoring, the process was not always a success. 'I try to ask them about the things they like,' said one subject. 'Question after question, to keep conversation going, but sometimes it doesn't work and they leave me.' This is hauntingly sad. After such a struggle to share human contact, it seems a doubly unjust blow.

The emotions of Aspergers when they are in a group are generally quite unlike those of the gregarious, and their behaviour can therefore seem very odd and sometimes alienating. I remember a night at the theatre with friends. After the show, we headed for the bar, where we turned our attention to the identity of various actors depicted in yellowing photographs hanging against the flock-papered walls. A nearby couple overheard our discussion and stepped in to give us some unasked-for information about a face we could not identify. At first, I felt extremely uncomfortable, then adrift and alone, but my gregarious friend introduced us. 'At this point,' he remembered, 'your face darkened, and friendly non-intrusive questions were met with blunt, unsmiling, monosyllabic replies which caused initial surprise, then obvious offence. I was as nonplussed as them by your behaviour but realised something was up so we drank up and left. Walking to the cab rank you got quite animated with me, asking, "How can you talk to those people? You don't even *know them*."'

Typical people are said to be like cooked spaghetti, soft and all mixed together, while Aspergers are more like uncooked spaghetti. If you try to bend them they snap. I have never been good in groups. Beyond two or three people I feel frightened, alone, and angry. This has landed me in all kinds of trouble, but trying to explain it to people has never got me very far. It is as hard as trying to tell a man who enjoys Brussels sprouts why and how you loathe them.

Let's say I am out to dinner with two or three people, or perhaps I am at a party for a family anniversary. This is how it feels:

I am a child of four and my parents have lost track of me in the busy central railway station of a frightening foreign country. Cutlery is being rattled and dropped, trains are whistling incessantly, there is loud unfamiliar music thumping in the background, and dogs are snarling. I am wearing somebody else's scratchy overcoat, which has something sticky on it, and there is in the place an overwhelming smell of turpentine, eggs, gas, and coal tar. The fluorescent lights are being turned on and off every second, and people keep grabbing my hand. Others are firing questions at me, incessantly demanding something, though I don't know what. I cannot tell whether they are friendly or dangerous. I don't understand the language and there is no way to explain myself. Everyone seems to know something I don't. They keep looking at one another. It is very cold or hot. Someone is screaming, sweat is trickling down my ribcage, and everything is buzzing. 'Cheer up; it might never 'appen,' says a disembodied voice over my shoulder. I look about desperately for anything I recognise but I am lost, my heart is in my mouth, and I feel as if I might faint. I cannot make sense of any of it, so I close in on myself, stare vacantly into the distance, looking aloof and unfriendly. I stop responding. I shut down.

This is how it is for me. For others it will be different.

★

After Kanner and Asperger, the next big name to appear on the international autism scene was another Austrian, Bruno Bettelheim (1903–1990). For three decades he was director of the Orthogenic School for Disturbed Children, in Chicago, where he cultivated an international reputation as a world expert in the psychotherapeutic treatment of autism, which he believed has a psychological cause.

In his 1967 volume, *The Empty Fortress: infantile autism and the birth of the self,* Bettelheim popularised Leo Kanner's original 'refrigerator' mothers idea — later rejected by Kanner — which proposed that autistic children were the victims of parental coldness, having been 'left neatly in refrigerators which did not defrost'.

In 1972, psychiatrist Dr Marian DeMyer, of Indiana University, decided to test the idea in a vigilant, properly done trial. Comparing the parents of a wide group of ordinary as well as autistic children she found there was nothing in their behaviour to tell them apart: the theory appeared to be false. But to Bettelheim, who had always viewed science with a jaundiced eye, this was water off a duck's back. He refused to admit that all advances in the understanding of the complex biological and environmental influences on the development of autism have been scientific. The psychoanalytic approach has got us nowhere.

Though Bruno Bettelheim's church had been shown to be built on sand, there was worse to come. In 1990, the year of his death,

Charles Pekow, a sometime resident of Bettelheim's illustrious school, wrote a withering article for The *Washington Post*, in which he described having seen Bettelheim drag children across the floor by their hair. A second former inmate spoke of living for years 'in abject, animal terror', while another said that Bettelheim had once pulled her out of the shower and beaten her, wet and naked, in front of a room full of people. 'To put it plainly,' remarked Leo Kanner's colleague Leon Eisenberg, 'he was a sadistic monster and doesn't deserve serious treatment as a scientist.'

★

In the 1950s, autism was believed to affect just four or five people in every ten thousand, but the inclusion of those with Asperger's syndrome, and the growing awareness of the condition, has caused an inevitable rise in recorded figures. Estimates vary between countries, depending on how the cake is cut, but The National Autistic Society says that today autism is reckoned in the UK to occur in more than one in every hundred people. The UN recently estimated the UK population to be 66,573,504. One per cent of this strangely precise number is about 665,000 autistic people. The NAS estimate is 700,000.

The broadening of criteria and increase in diagnoses has caused some opportunistic characters to promote noxious or useless treatments, while still others have identified environmental causes that are not actually there. The result has been the popularisation of a good deal of harmful claptrap dressed up as science.

In February 1998 the august medical journal the *Lancet* published a remarkable paper by gastroenterologist and medical researcher Dr Andrew Wakefield, which he had written with twelve colleagues. The paper said that shortly after receiving the triple MMR (measles, mumps, rubella) vaccine, eight out of twelve children that Wakefield had studied had developed bowel problems and signs of autism. This was big news, as the MMR vaccine had been used safely around the world for decades.

In a press conference, Wakefield urged parents to give their children yearly single vaccinations instead of the MMR, in case the triple jab might be too much for some children's immune systems. Flying in the face of accepted medical advice, as it did, this caused a worldwide news storm. Parents were understandably alarmed, and some decided not to give their children any jabs at all, causing a marked drop-off in vaccination rates, and a longer-term rise in measles cases.

Despite many clinicians expressing doubts about his paper Dr Wakefield continued to defend it. However, a robust British Medical Association study, which examined research from a hundred and eighty countries, eventually found no evidence for the proposition that the MMR jab was associated either with autism or inflammatory bowel disease.

Ten of the study's twelve co-authors finally disowned its conclusions, and the *Lancet* announced that it was retracting the 1998 paper. In January 2010, twelve years after Wakefield's initial report, Britain's General Medical Council called his work 'irresponsible' and 'dishonest'. The *British Medical Journal* said the whole fiasco was 'an elaborate fraud', and Dr Wakefield was struck off the medical register.

Although Andrew Wakefield's findings could not be, and never were, repeated by others, he has long continued to reject all the criticisms made about him, and despite repeated studies exonerating the MMR jab from any link with autism, a survey revealed that ten years after the first doubts were raised a quarter of Americans still believed that the triple vaccine could cause autism. There again, a 2011 Associated Press–GfK poll showed that more than three-quarters of them believed that angels are real. Research into autism, its causes, and its fascinatingly mysterious nature deserves better than wishful thinking, dishonesty, and wilful ignorance.

Many treatments for autism have been tried over the years, including special diets, various drugs, and, one suspects, more best-quality snake oil. Almost all have proved entirely useless. People have tried wrapping autistics in wet towels, burying them up to their necks in sand, and, of course, a range of Freudian whimsies. One Swiss parent wondered whether his son's condition might have been occasioned by his grandfather having gone to bed with a nun.

What is needed here is proper scientific investigation, not hopeless piffle like this. The research field is vast, ranging from the science of the brain, to social behaviour, to the huge variety of presenting profiles across the spectrum, from the speechless, intellectually impaired epileptic girl who bites her mother and cannot look after herself, to the brilliant oddballs in the Asperger's part of the spectrum: the strange but dazzling film director, the weird but inspired interpreter of Bach on the piano, or the very odd, focused, and incredibly brainy politician.

A remarkable case of success in the arts coupled with social imagination problems and late diagnosis of Asperger's is nicely illustrated by the case of the boy from a smoky Welsh steel town who became a Hollywood actor.

Anthony 'Tony' Hopkins was born on New Year's Eve 1937, in a suburb of Port Talbot, an industrial seaside town on the eastern margin of Swansea Bay. 'I was a poor learner,' he says, 'which left me open to ridicule and gave me an inferiority complex … I grew up absolutely convinced I was stupid.' He told Franz Lidz of the *New York Times* that he was 'an angry, unsettled boy full of rage' and that he'd had a 'useless and thoroughly confusing childhood'. 'I couldn't understand what everybody was talking about,' he said. Much of this rings bells with me.

In a 2017 interview with Bruce Fessier of the *Desert Sun*, Hopkins mentioned in passing that he had been diagnosed in his seventies with Asperger's syndrome. To many people this must have sounded implausible. How could this successful, articulate, witty man, who looked and seemed perfectly normal, be autistic?

Hopkins describes himself as a 'high end' Asperger, meaning that his distinctive troubles and their cause were not immediately apparent under the gloss of 'normality' and professional success. Even so, his underlying problems are classically autistic.

He was a very isolated child who was never really close to anyone, and for the most part this has lasted into adulthood. 'I don't have many friends,' he says, 'I'm very much a loner … I don't go to parties.'

Having failed to shine academically, Anthony Hopkins sought refuge in painting and drawing. He was also a very good pianist. He says that if he had been 'clever enough' he would have gone to music college. 'As it was,' he continues, 'I had to settle for being an actor.'

He studied at the Royal Academy of Dramatic Art in London before earning a crust in a repertory company, where he was spotted by Laurence Olivier, who asked him to join the National Theatre.

Perhaps inevitably, Hopkins never fitted in with the theatrical establishment. 'I was never sure what the hell I was,' he said. 'That led to years of deep insecurity and curiosity. I could never settle anywhere. I was troubled and caused trouble, especially in my early years.' Though I have never caused trouble — at least not on purpose — this sums up the way I felt as a young man.

Hopkins got on more happily in films, his portrayal of serial killer Hannibal Lecter in *The Silence of the Lambs* (1991) earning him great popular acclaim. On seeing the film his mother reportedly told him, 'I always knew you were strange.'

As well as strangeness, Anthony Hopkins has been blessed with some other remarkable endowments. He is a good composer and has written his own film music. When John Crace of *The Guardian* asked him what kind of conductor he might have made he replied, 'One who knew the names of every member of the orchestra ...'

His phenomenal memory is well known in the film business. In Steven Spielberg's *Amistad* Hopkins astounded director and crew with his one-take, word-perfect performance of a seven-page monologue.

You might object that any stage actor would be used to memorising lengthy speeches, but Hopkins' memory is more curious than this. For example, he has a great facility for recalling times and dates. Gaby Wood, interviewing him for *The Guardian* in 1998, remarked that he was, 'an addict of detail' and referred to his 'intricate, rigorous method' and his 'rigid control'.

Rigid control and attention to detail are attributes typical of Aspergers, who are, for instance, often consumed by their need to keep good time. Anthony Hopkins is always crisply punctual. This too we have in common.

Among his other interests are painting, driving alone in his car for thousands of miles at a time, and watching the same *Carry On* films and Tommy Cooper shows over and over.

On casting him in his 1995 film *Nixon*, Oliver Stone said he had noticed Hopkins' 'aloneness' and wanted him for that reason. In using the word employed by Leo Kanner to characterise his autistic boys half a century before, Stone was homing in on something central to Hopkins' human makeup.

He was perfectly cast in *The Remains of the Day* (1993) as an apparently unempathic, diffident, buttoned up, rigid, rule-mad, fastidious, pedantic butler, a man who, when the woman he secretly loves offers to put flowers in his room, says flatly, 'I prefer to keep things as they are.'

Hopkins was once a heavy drinker, but he no longer drinks and has mellowed since his troublesome youth. Perhaps finding his niche has done it. Life as a square peg in a series of round holes is enough to make anyone tense, and with understanding comes acceptance. 'I don't feel that awful kind of angst — like I was on the wrong planet — that I felt for years. I feel now I belong somewhere. I belong in my own skin ... It's a solitary life, but I love it.' This is a cheering message for anyone with Asperger's syndrome.

★

I look up from my bulging folder of notes as Sarah comes back into the room with a sheet of paper. The weather being pleasant, one of the windows in her office has been open since I sat down, the breeze stirring the curtain from time to time. All at once there is a noise, and from the corner of my eye I spot a sharp movement. A starling is standing on the tabletop: dark with white speckles and a beady eye. A mane of iridescent feathers shimmers in a rainbow of greasy blues, greens, and purples, contrasting with its dusky plumes below. Finding itself in unexpected company, the creature is as surprised as we are. It stands alert, with talons spread, taking in the situation.

Being closer than Sarah, I rise slowly from the seat, the folder in my hand. I have a vague idea that I will shoo the animal out of the window, but as I approach it starts in alarm, takes off, and settles on the cornice of the bookcase.

Without a word, Sarah extends an empty box file. Taking the file, I creep towards the starling, expecting it at any moment to fly from its perch back to the table. We could be here all day. But, as I close in, the bird sags resignedly and I drop the open box file over it, sliding the folder underneath. Sarah has the window open wide and is holding aside the curtain. Gingerly lifting the apparatus, I cross the room and reach out into the fresh air, lifting off the folder. But the bird just blinks at the vista without moving. 'Go on bird,' I say encouragingly, 'Fly!'

'Fly away bird,' says Sarah.

With a sudden blink, the animal launches itself into the fresh air and is away, free. I close the box file. On the spine I see the word, 'ASPERGER'S'.

'We're a great team,' I say.

'You did it all yourself,' says Sarah.

Before the meeting she had asked me to fill in a couple of questionnaires. The first is known as the Autism-Spectrum Quotient or just Autism Quotient (AQ). Together with evidence gathered from an interview, and from family members if possible, the questionnaires form the Adult Asperger Assessment (AAA).

The Adult Asperger Assessment and the Autism Quotient were both developed by Professor Simon Baron-Cohen and his team at Cambridge University's Autism Research Centre. The AQ is a short, easy-to-complete test, which anyone of average intelligence can do themselves in minutes. It was developed in the nineties and took off in 2001 after it was published in the technology magazine *Wired*, alongside an article amusingly entitled, 'The Geek Syndrome'. This headline is, like many headlines, somewhat misleading, since not everybody with Asperger's fits the geek stereotype, though perhaps more than a few of *Wired*'s editors and readers do.

The AQ is designed to measure the extent of autistic traits in adults — there are versions especially for children — and its fifty questions examine five particular areas: social skills, communication skills, social imagination, attention to detail, and attention switching (tolerance of change). These are areas in which the autistic brain tends to perform differently from the more typical brain.

For all its simplicity the test has been found to be a reliable indicator of autistic traits and is now widely used, sometimes as a self-test by people wanting a quick confirmation of something they have long suspected. The Autism Research Centre's website takes pains, however, to point out that the AQ was designed to be a descriptive rather than a diagnostic measure, warning that none of its test scores on their own will positively identify autism. People who are concerned or who need advice are recommended to talk to their family doctor or, in the UK, the National Autistic Society. I guess that a certain amount of this qualification may be, to use a technical legal term, 'arse covering'.

Here below is what the AQ looks like. It contains fifty forced-choice questions. You must tick one box for each question. There is no time limit, and if you would like to take the test yourself, the scoring method appears at the foot.

1. I prefer to do things with others rather than on my own.
    ☐ Definitely agree   ☐ Slightly agree   ☐ Slightly disagree   ☐ Definitely disagree

2. I prefer to do things the same way over and over again.
    ☐ Definitely agree   ☐ Slightly agree   ☐ Slightly disagree   ☐ Definitely disagree

3. If I try to imagine something, I find it very easy to create a picture in my mind.

   ☐ Definitely agree   ☐ Slightly agree   ☐ Slightly disagree   ☐ Definitely disagree

4. I frequently get so strongly absorbed in one thing that I lose sight of other things.

   ☐ Definitely agree   ☐ Slightly agree   ☐ Slightly disagree   ☐ Definitely disagree

5. I often notice small sounds when others do not.

   ☐ Definitely agree   ☐ Slightly agree   ☐ Slightly disagree   ☐ Definitely disagree

6. I usually notice car number plates or similar strings of information.

   ☐ Definitely agree   ☐ Slightly agree   ☐ Slightly disagree   ☐ Definitely disagree

7. Other people frequently tell me that what I've said is impolite, even though I think it is polite.

   ☐ Definitely agree   ☐ Slightly agree   ☐ Slightly disagree   ☐ Definitely disagree

8. When I'm reading a story, I can easily imagine what the characters might look like.

   ☐ Definitely agree   ☐ Slightly agree   ☐ Slightly disagree   ☐ Definitely disagree

9. I am fascinated by dates.

   ☐ Definitely agree   ☐ Slightly agree   ☐ Slightly disagree   ☐ Definitely disagree

10. In a social group, I can easily keep track of several different people's conversations.

   ☐ Definitely agree   ☐ Slightly agree   ☐ Slightly disagree   ☐ Definitely disagree

11. I find social situations easy.

   ☐ Definitely agree   ☐ Slightly agree   ☐ Slightly disagree   ☐ Definitely disagree

12. I tend to notice details that others do not.

☐ Definitely agree   ☐ Slightly agree   ☐ Slightly disagree   ☐ Definitely disagree

13. I would rather go to a library than to a party.

☐ Definitely agree   ☐ Slightly agree   ☐ Slightly disagree   ☐ Definitely disagree

14. I find making up stories easy.

☐ Definitely agree   ☐ Slightly agree   ☐ Slightly disagree   ☐ Definitely disagree

15. I find myself drawn more strongly to people than to things.

☐ Definitely agree   ☐ Slightly agree   ☐ Slightly disagree   ☐ Definitely disagree

16. I tend to have very strong interests, which I get upset about if I can't pursue.

☐ Definitely agree   ☐ Slightly agree   ☐ Slightly disagree   ☐ Definitely disagree

17. I enjoy social chitchat.

☐ Definitely agree   ☐ Slightly agree   ☐ Slightly disagree   ☐ Definitely disagree

18. When I talk, it isn't always easy for others to get a word in edgewise.

☐ Definitely agree   ☐ Slightly agree   ☐ Slightly disagree   ☐ Definitely disagree

19. I am fascinated by numbers.

☐ Definitely agree   ☐ Slightly agree   ☐ Slightly disagree   ☐ Definitely disagree

20. When I'm reading a story, I find it difficult to work out the characters' intentions.

☐ Definitely agree   ☐ Slightly agree   ☐ Slightly disagree   ☐ Definitely disagree

21. I don't particularly enjoy reading fiction.

☐ Definitely agree   ☐ Slightly agree   ☐ Slightly disagree   ☐ Definitely disagree

22. I find it hard to make new friends.

☐ Definitely agree ☐ Slightly agree ☐ Slightly disagree ☐ Definitely disagree

23. I notice patterns in things all the time.

☐ Definitely agree ☐ Slightly agree ☐ Slightly disagree ☐ Definitely disagree

24. I would rather go to the theatre than to a museum.

☐ Definitely agree ☐ Slightly agree ☐ Slightly disagree ☐ Definitely disagree

25. It does not upset me if my daily routine is disturbed.

☐ Definitely agree ☐ Slightly agree ☐ Slightly disagree ☐ Definitely disagree

26. I frequently find that I don't know how to keep a conversation going.

☐ Definitely agree ☐ Slightly agree ☐ Slightly disagree ☐ Definitely disagree

27. I find it easy to 'read between the lines' when someone is talking to me.

☐ Definitely agree ☐ Slightly agree ☐ Slightly disagree ☐ Definitely disagree

28. I usually concentrate more on the whole picture, rather than on the small details.

☐ Definitely agree ☐ Slightly agree ☐ Slightly disagree ☐ Definitely disagree

29. I am not very good at remembering phone numbers.

☐ Definitely agree ☐ Slightly agree ☐ Slightly disagree ☐ Definitely disagree

30. I don't usually notice small changes in a situation or a person's appearance.

☐ Definitely agree ☐ Slightly agree ☐ Slightly disagree ☐ Definitely disagree

31. I know how to tell if someone listening to me is getting bored.

☐ Definitely agree ☐ Slightly agree ☐ Slightly disagree ☐ Definitely disagree

32. I find it easy to do more than one thing at once.

   ☐ Definitely agree   ☐ Slightly agree   ☐ Slightly disagree   ☐ Definitely disagree

33. When I talk on the phone, I'm not sure when it's my turn to speak.

   ☐ Definitely agree   ☐ Slightly agree   ☐ Slightly disagree   ☐ Definitely disagree

34. I enjoy doing things spontaneously.

   ☐ Definitely agree   ☐ Slightly agree   ☐ Slightly disagree   ☐ Definitely disagree

35. I am often the last to understand the point of a joke.

   ☐ Definitely agree   ☐ Slightly agree   ☐ Slightly disagree   ☐ Definitely disagree

36. I find it easy to work out what someone is thinking or feeling just by looking at their face.

   ☐ Definitely agree   ☐ Slightly agree   ☐ Slightly disagree   ☐ Definitely disagree

37. If there is an interruption, I can switch back to what I was doing very quickly.

   ☐ Definitely agree   ☐ Slightly agree   ☐ Slightly disagree   ☐ Definitely disagree

38. I am good at social chitchat.

   ☐ Definitely agree   ☐ Slightly agree   ☐ Slightly disagree   ☐ Definitely disagree

39. People often tell me that I keep going on and on about the same thing.

   ☐ Definitely agree   ☐ Slightly agree   ☐ Slightly disagree   ☐ Definitely disagree

40. When I was young, I used to enjoy playing games involving pretending with other children.

   ☐ Definitely agree   ☐ Slightly agree   ☐ Slightly disagree   ☐ Definitely disagree

41. I like to collect information about categories of things (e.g. types of cars, birds, trains, plants).

   ☐ Definitely agree   ☐ Slightly agree   ☐ Slightly disagree   ☐ Definitely disagree

42. I find it difficult to imagine what it would be like to be someone else.

☐ Definitely agree   ☐ Slightly agree   ☐ Slightly disagree   ☐ Definitely disagree

43. I like to carefully plan any activities I participate in.

☐ Definitely agree   ☐ Slightly agree   ☐ Slightly disagree   ☐ Definitely disagree

44. I enjoy social occasions.

☐ Definitely agree   ☐ Slightly agree   ☐ Slightly disagree   ☐ Definitely disagree

45. I find it difficult to work out people's intentions.

☐ Definitely agree   ☐ Slightly agree   ☐ Slightly disagree   ☐ Definitely disagree

46. New situations make me anxious.

☐ Definitely agree   ☐ Slightly agree   ☐ Slightly disagree   ☐ Definitely disagree

47. I enjoy meeting new people.

☐ Definitely agree   ☐ Slightly agree   ☐ Slightly disagree   ☐ Definitely disagree

48. I am a good diplomat.

☐ Definitely agree   ☐ Slightly agree   ☐ Slightly disagree   ☐ Definitely disagree

49. I am not very good at remembering people's date of birth.

☐ Definitely agree   ☐ Slightly agree   ☐ Slightly disagree   ☐ Definitely disagree

50. I find it very easy to play games with children that involve pretending.

☐ Definitely agree   ☐ Slightly agree   ☐ Slightly disagree   ☐ Definitely disagree

SOURCE: AUTISM RESEARCH CENTRE

Scoring

- Score 1 point per question if you ticked 'Definitely agree' or 'Slightly agree' for questions 2, 4, 5, 6, 7, 9, 12, 13, 16, 18, 19, 20, 21, 22, 23, 26, 33, 35, 39, 41, 42, 43, 45, and 46.
- Score 1 point per question if you ticked 'Definitely disagree' or 'Slightly disagree' for questions 1, 3, 8, 10, 11, 14, 15, 17, 24, 25, 27, 28, 29, 30, 31, 32, 34, 36, 37, 38, 40, 44, 47, 48, 49, and 50.
- For a final result, add up the total number of points you have scored.

Nobody really scores zero on the Autism Quotient. Everybody has some autistic traits. But this does not mean that everybody is 'a bit autistic'. The average (mean) AQ score for non-autistic people is about 17, with men typically scoring a couple of points higher than women. But the great majority of average intelligence Aspergers score 32 or more, indicating clinically significant levels of autistic traits. A score of less than 26 effectively rules out Asperger's syndrome.

If you score highly on the test, other members of your family — parents, brothers, sisters, children — are also likely to score highly. There is genetic evidence that some (though not all) parents of autistic children exhibit the same autism traits as their offspring, though to a milder degree. This sub-autistic group is referred to by the off-putting technical name 'broader autism phenotype' or BAP. The BAP is a cloud of people sharing autistic attributes in common, who don't score high enough on the AQ to win an autism diagnosis. In any case, the presence of just one person in the family having autism greatly increases the likelihood of somebody else in the family also having it.

The exact male-to-female ratio for autism and Asperger's

syndrome in the general population is the subject of much debate. For classic autism, it is commonly said to be four males for every female, with the ratio for Asperger's syndrome being much higher, at nine males to every female, though there is good evidence that, in girls and women, autism, including Asperger's, is routinely missed because they express it differently. For example, female Aspergers seem to be better at blending in and camouflaging their autistic traits. Perhaps one day the number of diagnosed girls and women will equal the number of boys and men.

In the evolutionary past, when our cavewomen ancestors were multi-tasking, cuddling babies, chopping radishes, and organising the village between themselves, caveman behaviour such as going off with some other blokes in search of dinner, with a couple of good spears designed and made by themselves, was no doubt useful. An ability to spot the movement of a deer in the brush and hit it without being distracted by social chitchat would have been a useful talent. Today, when we hunt our food not on the savannah but in the supermarket, and don't need to build a bridge over every stream we encounter, such typically male skills as single-mindedness and attention to systems have been usefully shifted to fields such as engineering and science.

Hans Asperger noted that the children he had studied tended to have a gift for logic and scientific observation. Precise thinking and formulating were so highly developed in them, he said, that their relationship to other people had been 'lost'. 'For success in science,' he remarked, 'a dash of autism is essential'.

To test the idea that there is a genetic association between scientific and mathematical aptitude, technical intelligence, and the risk of autism in offspring, Simon Baron-Cohen decided to look at a town with a concentration of nerdy occupations. Choosing

Eindhoven, Holland's Silicon Valley, where a third of jobs are in IT, he found the rate of child autism to be more than twice that of Haarlem or Utrecht, towns with comparable demographics but no concentration of IT jobs. The clear inference was that the high rate of technical occupations among parents was associated with an increased likelihood of autism in offspring.

Baron-Cohen also discovered that an unusually high number of autistic children had fathers and grandfathers, on both sides of the family, who were engineers. Like having an intense interest in trains, having a parent or grandparent who was an engineer seems to be a badge that indicates an increased likelihood of autism.

It is often said that, along with their preoccupation with technology, systems, engineering, and science, people with Asperger's syndrome do not feel empathy. Dr Watson describes his friend Sherlock Holmes as 'an isolated phenomenon, a brain without a heart, as deficient in human sympathy as he was pre-eminent in intelligence …' This is a perfect description of the Asperger's aloof and seemingly unempathic detachment.

The definition of 'empathy' in Oxford's online dictionary is 'the ability to understand and share the feelings of another', and if you are judged to lack this quality you are viewed as missing something essentially human. The parable of the Good Samaritan embodies the essence of empathy.

Empathy may be sorted into two kinds: cognitive (intellectual) and affective (emotional). Cognitive empathy is the ability to understand the feelings of others, and is related to the theory of mind. Affective empathy is quite different: it is the sensibility aroused by someone's suffering, and the consequent desire to help. Psychopaths are experts in cognitive empathy, understanding how a person is feeling and why, but lacking in affective empathy. They are not touched. This is why they can lie persuasively, often with great charm, or be coldly cruel and manipulative.

Unlike psychopaths, autistics have trouble with cognitive empathy, and find it difficult to understand the reasons for another person's feelings. They are confused by people and may unwittingly say harsh things or give their undiluted opinion without grasping that this might be hurtful. If chided they may miss the point and object that what they are saying is true. Their affective empathy, however, is intact. They feel sadness at someone's suffering. They become upset, show concern, and wish to help, and they often have a very strong moral conscience.

A genetic contribution to the trait of empathy was demonstrated in a striking piece of research published by the Autism Research Centre in 2013. The study linked a particular gene, the forgettably named GABRB3 gene, not only to empathy but also to Asperger's syndrome. The team described abnormal social behaviour in GABRB3-deficient mice. Unlike control mice with normal GABRB3, the affected mice tended to avoid contact when introduced to a stranger mouse. They also demonstrated repetitive behaviour, thus displaying two core traits needed for a (human) diagnosis of an autism spectrum condition. When the studies were extended to humans with Asperger's syndrome they confirmed that variations in GABRB3 are connected with differences in empathy and Asperger's syndrome alike.

Despite these findings, some people with Asperger's syndrome maintain that it is non-autistics who are truly unempathic. People with more typical brains often fail to understand, or make any effort to understand, how Aspergers feel or why they are behaving in certain ways. At school and at work Aspergers routinely put up with a good deal of cold-blooded, unempathic, and unkind treatment.

To measure empathy in adults, the ARC devised a questionnaire — the Empathy Quotient (EQ) — that resembles the Autism Quotient. Overall, women score higher on the EQ than do men. Autistics, male and female, score lower than typical people.

The team at the ARC compared and contrasted empathy with the complementary trait of 'systemisation', which is the analysis of systems in search of the underlying canons that govern them. They confirmed that the average male brain is better at understanding and constructing systems and less empathic. The average female brain, is, by contrast, less good at systemising and is more social and more empathic. People with autism, both male and female, likewise show a stronger interest in systems, a predilection that had been noted from the earliest days. Systems might be mechanical, like the car engine, they might be natural, like the weather, or organisational, like a library. People with autism, along with scientists, love to systemise.

The way autistics see the world and process information resembles the way in which scientists routinely think. This does not mean that autistics do better in science exams or become scientists. It is more to do with the way they look at the world. Science questions, like philosophy questions, are often childishly simple: Why is ice slippery? Why is there something and not nothing? Why did that apple fall downwards? Such apparently naive questions can quickly lead to complex answers about the deep nature of reality.

Autistics, including Aspergers, commonly like things to be highly structured and neatly categorised, and can become fascinated by patterns and the underlying rules that govern systems. The autistic mind is one, says Simon Baron-Cohen, which is striving 'to set aside the temporal dimension in order to see — in stark relief — the eternal repeating patterns in nature'.

The ARC team tried to give a united explanation of the two essential, but different, autistic traits — the social and communication difficulties (empathy problems) and the narrow interests and attention to detail (systemising and analytical aptitude). They called their idea the empathising–systemising (E–S) theory. Their method allows everybody who completes a questionnaire — whether autistic or not — to be plotted as a dot somewhere on a scatter plot, based on their combination of systemising and empathising characteristics.

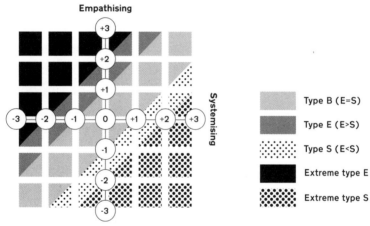

SOURCE: AUTISM RESEARCH CENTRE

Along the vertical axis is empathy, which goes from -3 to +3. Zero is the average for the population. Above zero you are better than average at reading thoughts and feelings and responding with appropriate emotion. Below zero you have increasing problems. The horizontal axis represents systemising. To the right of zero you are better than average at understanding and creating systems. To the left of zero you are decreasingly good. The idea of this simple graph is that *everybody* falls somewhere in the space.

As expected, the results show that more women than men fall in the top, narrow diagonal strip (Type E: empathising), their empathy tending to be greater than their systemising. In the pale wide diagonal across the centre (Type B: balanced), subjects are equally good, or bad, with empathy and with systems. The lowermost diagonal strip (Type S: systemising) is where more men fall, with systemising ability generally higher than empathising.

The expectation was that autistic people, who are naturally drawn to the predicable systemised world rather than the 'less lawful' and unpredictable world of people, would fall somewhere in the lower-right corner of the bottom-right triangle, with systemising anywhere from average to above average, but empathy at less than minus one and consequent problems with human relationships. And so it proved. Male and female autistics clustered in this part of the diagram (Extreme Type S).

Although there has been criticism of the E–S theory from various quarters, the diagram surely confirms what everybody already knew — that many more web developers and sewer engineers are men, and more nursery school teachers and receptionists are women. Is it any wonder that in jobs such as nursing, waiting on tables, and serving passengers in aeroplanes, where empathy is a basic essential, it is mainly women who are employed? In experiments, female monkeys prefer to play with dolls than with toy trains, while male monkeys do the opposite. So it's not (merely) a question of gender stereotyping. Simon Baron-Cohen says it should come as no surprise, since males and females differ below the neck, that we should find some differences above the neck too.

This is not to say that nature has everything and nurture nothing to do with the work we all end up doing, or that there isn't still a strong bias in some places, including the home, towards the idea that boys and men ought to do certain things only, and girls and women others.

In 2015 an English biochemist named Tim Hunt told a conference about his trouble with allowing 'girls' to be in the same science lab as men. He said: 'You fall in love with them, they fall in love with you, and when you criticise them, they cry.' This attitude was angrily denounced by a few, though most people I spoke to, men and women alike, just laughed. Amusement is the proper response to such muttonheaded dottiness.

Unhappily, the whole area of sexual differences in career choice is emotionally fraught, and our understanding of the complexities of why we do what we do, is still in its infancy. We do know, however, that men tend to be more solitary, terser, more systematically and mechanically minded, and more inclined to try to solve their own problems. More men than women kill themselves, and more men have Asperger's diagnoses.

But, though there are more male autistics than female, this is not essentially a matter of sex. In fact, the E–S theory is a better predictor than your genitals of whether you will choose to study STEM subjects (Science, Technology, Engineering, and Mathematics). What has been positively selected in evolutionary terms, Simon Baron-Cohen believes, is not autism itself, but an aptitude for understanding or building systems, including mathematics.

He explored the idea of a link between autism and 'maleness' in what he has termed 'the extreme male brain theory' of autism, for which he says there are biological reasons. Brain differences are apparent from the earliest days, and there is evidence, he believes, that the seeds are sown before birth.

Males produce twice as much testosterone as females, and it is high levels of testosterone in the womb, he says, not whether you are male or female, which seems to be related to autism and scientific talent alike; testosterone present in the foetus shapes brain development and plays a role also in influencing both empathising and systemising. Whether you are male or female, elevated levels of pre-natal testosterone are associated with more autistic traits, including a greater interest in systems and less eye contact at the age of one. Babies who stare much more at a geometric mobile than at a human face tend to go on to develop autism.

Although the extreme male brain theory is a persuasive way of looking at the place of the complementary traits of sytemising and empathising in autistics and society as a whole, it has not gone down well with feminist critics, some of whom point out that a more pertinent example of a person with an extreme male brain would be a football hooligan. But this is just jolly wordplay.

Psychologist Professor Cordelia Fine is a member of something called the NeuroGenderings Network, described as 'a transdisciplinary network of "neurofeminist" scholars who aim to critically examine neuroscientific knowledge production and to develop differentiated approaches for a more gender-adequate neuroscientific research'. Fine referred to Baron-Cohen's findings as an example of 'neurosexism'. I'm not sure what 'knowledge production' is, but if Professor Fine doesn't believe that women and girls are self-evidently more sociable than men and boys I think she should get out more.

The National Autistic Society's Lorna Wing Centre for Autism says it has seen a steady increase in the number of girls and women referred for diagnosis, which, it says, suggests a historic bias towards men and boys in the criteria that are used. Whether this is a male-chauvinist-pig bias by a lot of sexist autism specialists who won't allow women to join their gentlemen's club, or the sort of bias that means more men than women get testicle cancer, who can say? Whatever the case, there just are significantly more male autistics diagnosed than female. How many woman trainspotters do you know? This does not mean, however, that more work should not be done to identify and help those many autistic girls and women who have been, and continue to be, missed.

The 'extreme male brain' type is present not only in computer nerds and cartographers, it also extends to such systems as languages, medicine, and politics, which is highly systematic, being a system of administrative and organisational rules resting on an underlying system of beliefs and moral principles.

★

In the latter half of the twentieth century, two English politicians, who were both, probably not coincidentally, members of 'the awkward squad' showed clear traits of Asperger's syndrome.

For half a century, between 1950 and 2001, Tony Benn (1925–2014) was a Labour Member of Parliament. Among the government jobs he held were Postmaster General, and Minister of Technology.

In 1960, on the death of his father Lord Stansgate, Benn inherited a peerage he didn't want because it disallowed him from continuing as an MP. He successfully campaigned to renounce the title and got the law changed so that he could carry on in the House of Commons.

In typical Asperger style, Tony Benn's personal, political, and moral convictions were deeply held, and he said that he had 'a very strong sense of right and wrong'. One of his repeated dictums was that you should say what you mean and mean what you say, and he explained that he would not want to be in politics if he was dancing to somebody else's tune. He stuck to his opinions through thick and thin, telling *Socialist Review* in 2007: 'I would be ashamed if I thought I'd ever said anything I didn't believe to get on.'

Benn was completely unimpressed by authority, for which he had a profound distaste. At the age of five or six he was taken out of Bible class for interjecting his own opinions. Interference incensed him and he had 'a deep suspicion of being bullied and lectured and harassed ... by people who claim to have some authority over you'. Once wanting to smoke his pipe on a train he peeled the no-smoking sticker off the window in an act of civil disobedience and personal fury.

When he was a minister he was frequently attacked in the press. He took this with some aplomb but could never grasp why the tabloids, as well as criticising his opinions, wrote untrue things about him. Deliberate untruth seemed to mystify him. Interviewed by Dr Anthony Clare for BBC Radio 4's *In the Psychiatrist's Chair*, in 1995, he explained: 'To begin with I didn't quite understand why they should say such absurd things.' The preference for plain truth and difficulty in accepting that people dissemble and lie is typical of Aspergers.

Though decently turned out in the Chamber and on television, Benn could sometimes look slightly odd, having a preference for pale brown shoes with a Velcro flap, the colour and folksy informality of which clashed with the propriety of the sober suits and jackets he favoured.

His tastes in food were faddish. He was an almost obsessive fan of tea, drinking pints of it throughout the day, and mentioning it frequently in interviews. He drank no alcohol, and in his forties became a vegetarian, having decided to avoid both booze and burgers on moral grounds. Lunch was almost always a pizza, a banana, and more tea. Along with the cluster of other intriguing traits, this amusing food and drink fad was suggestive.

Benn's life was rigidly routine: he said that he went to bed at twenty-five to one every night and got up at five to seven. 'I find it very difficult to go to bed if I haven't done my diary,' he explained. His diary keeping was as obsessive as his tea drinking.

Even as a child, structure, ritual, and routine had been important to him. He was obsessed with time and time keeping, and he kept account books of his pocket money. 'Temperance, and tea, and accounts, and time have been very much a part of the framework of my life,' he told Clare, 'and in a way, once you've got all that straight you're free to get on with your life … so it's quite comforting to have a reasonable structure.' This is something that any Asperger would understand.

He described himself as 'a gregarious soul', but his attitude to other people was odd. At the end of one short television interview he seemed discombobulated by the interviewer's extended hand. The resulting handshake looked very weird.

The ability to process emotion and deal with it in a standard way eludes many Aspergers. Tony Benn was a highly emotional man, who was easily moved by the suffering of others and shed tears in the House of Commons. His elder brother was killed in the Second World War and he was permanently and deeply affected by this loss. He frequently mentioned this brother, and the bereavement seemed unusually fresh in his mind even towards the end of his long life.

As minister of technology, with a hi-tech remit, Benn was ideally cast. He was a technology nerd with what he called 'a nostalgic love of steam' and a fascination for gadgetry of all kinds, including digital watches that did all sorts of other things, and a series of his own string-and-sticky-tape inventions. He recorded all his media interviews on the latest equipment to check that what he said was accurately reported, and among his own mad-professor inventions were a car-mounted armchair, a plastic doohickey for holding a lot of pens in his pocket, and a briefcase that turned into a lectern for public speaking. This last device prefigured his most commercial contraption.

In 2010, at the age of eighty-five, Benn unveiled a suitcase he had invented with a fold-down canvas fisherman's stool attached. Having first called it the Backbencher, the safest seat in parliament, he renamed it the Seatcase.

This demonstration of focus, mechanics, gadgetry, and sedulous attention to detail shows why, perhaps, autistic traits have not died out with natural selection. They are extremely useful.

In his *Memoirs* (1991) novelist Kingsley Amis remembered meeting Tony Benn and also Benn's fellow MP Enoch Powell, of the Conservative Party. Amis thought he had discovered why neither had ever managed to lead his party, though each had come within a whisker of it: both men, he said, in typically rude style, 'looked barmy'.

Enoch Powell (1912–1998) was a very strange politician, with a rich portfolio of characteristics that very clearly suggest Asperger's syndrome.

A classicist, and languages expert, Powell was nicknamed 'the professor' as a child. One schoolfriend described him as 'fiendishly clever', intense and serious, and 'a complete loner'.

Simon Heffer, in *Like The Roman: the life of Enoch Powell* (1999), notes the following traits: aloofness, attention to detail, brusqueness, concentration, courtesy, frugality, good with children, intellectual arrogance, lack of warmth, rarely smiles, reclusiveness, refusal to compromise, remorseless logic, repressed emotions, reserve, risk-taking, romanticism, sense of absolutes, and solitariness. This diagnostic checklist of Asperger traits is quoted by Viktoria Lyons and Michael Fitzgerald in their 2005 book, *Asperger Syndrome — A Gift or a Curse?*

Tucked away in the list is a mention of Powell's ability to get on with children. So formal and upright was his demeanour that this gift seemed unlikely to some. But to see him, in a television documentary, talking to a toddler, it is quite clear that he loved children. And they loved him.

According to his biographer, Robert Shepherd, Powell was himself a 'serious minded and rather withdrawn child, who was happy always studying and seemed older than his years'. He was also the victim of what Shepherd called other children's 'mischief', in other words, teasing. His parents appeared 'rather remote' and his father had interests in mathematics and ornithology. His mother was uncommonly bright, but strange, teaching herself Greek, and dressing in old-fashioned costumes.

An accomplished musician, Powell played the clarinet. He also won all the school prizes for Classics, his obsessive nitpicking resulting in him endlessly searching the Greek texts for errors.

Having admitted to broadcaster Michael Cockerell that as a schoolboy he had behaved delinquently on trains, he was asked to recall the details. With characteristic Asperger's formality he immediately delivered the following perfectly formed, if over-dressed, sentence: 'I hesitate to remember the depredations which I helped to commit upon the rolling stock of the Midland Railway Company.'

After school Powell went to Cambridge University. 'I had no social life as an undergraduate,' he recalled, 'I got up at five. I knew nothing else to do but to work ...' So averse to social situations was he that he refused to attend dinner with the Master of Trinity, the first time anyone had done this. 'He did not seem to want to share his life,' said a fellow student. There was 'something lonely in him', remembered one former colleague. Powell himself said, 'I can never be lonely enough.'

He spoke very strangely in what was described as a 'hypnotic, metallic voice', and his gaze was stiff and peculiar. The sometime British Prime Minister Harold Macmillan disliked sitting opposite him, finding himself unable to bear 'those mad eyes staring at me a moment longer'.

During the Second World War, Enoch Powell volunteered for the army and was rapidly promoted from the rank of private to brigadier. He loved the systematic structures and routines of the military but was regarded as very peculiar. In the heat of the African summer he always wore a shirt and tie, with long drill trousers and boots, and a tailored military jacket, which he claimed kept up his morale. Suggesting a stroll, a fellow soldier was astonished when Powell kept going for thirteen hours.

Hardy Amies, later the Queen's dress designer, was a fellow intelligence officer cadet. Bright and cheerful, he was very different to the dour Powell, who nonetheless took Amies' obvious homo-sexuality in his stride, seeing it as nothing more than a matter for playful teasing. The two remained lifelong friends. Openness to difference and lack of judgmentalism are two of the most admirable traits of people with Asperger's syndrome.

Out of uniform Powell was always superbly dressed, in beauti-ful, dark three-piece suits, white pocket hankie, and gleaming black shoes. He wore a bristling military moustache from his youth until his death, and his hair was so efficiently primped that it sometimes looked solid. Intriguingly, his wife remarked that above all Powell hated his hair being washed. She described how his young daughters used to 'queue up outside the door to hear his screams because he made such a performance'. His daughter Susan put it plainly: 'He does not like water on his head.' This heightened sensory reaction is just typical of Asperger's syndrome.

Powell had a lifelong interest in languages. He studied Urdu at the School of Oriental Studies and was a professor of Ancient Greek by the age of twenty-five. He was an expert on, and expert in, several other languages, including Welsh and Portuguese. By the time of his death he was highly proficient in fourteen of them.

He was a Member of Parliament between 1950 and 1974, and Minister of Health between 1960 and 1963. His politics were of the Right but, like the self-determined radical Tony Benn, he was always the 'odd man out', as he put it, among fellow members of his party, promoting his own very strongly held but unusual political and moral views. He had almost no political friends.

Personal relationships are difficult enough, but the girlfriend and boyfriend business can be its own special torment for Aspergers. Reading aloud one of his own published poems, written for a young woman who had turned down his proposal of marriage, Powell could not quite make it through the verse, and began to weep. 'You mustn't put me in this situation in which I'm so overcome by emotion,' he objected. He agreed that first love is the most intense, and, he added, 'mysterious'. Even in old age this long-ago loss seemed excessively painful to him.

Powell was unlucky in love until well into middle age and it was not until he was thirty-nine that he married Pamela Wilson, a wonderfully upbeat, patient, and outgoing lady of great cheer, his opposite in many ways. She explained that half the time even she could not make out what was going on in his mind.

She noticed soon after their marriage that he had difficulty in recognising faces. Wonderfully direct and amused, she told Michael Cockerell that a month after their honeymoon she went to meet Powell in the Central Lobby of the House of Commons. She was astonished to see him going all the way round, looking for her amongst some other ladies, 'wondering which one he'd married and been on a honeymoon with'.

While she was about it, Powell's wife, who, like many partners of people with Asperger's, seemed to have saintly endowments, reminded her husband, 'You've always had trouble riding a bicycle.' Difficulty with motor control is another typical Asperger trait.

Enoch Powell seemed to use his intellectual gifts to disguise some of his social ineptitude, but he was never able to crack the social code. Kingsley Amis remembered meeting him for the first time with a small group. He noticed that Powell spoke as though he were addressing a public meeting, but found him agreeable enough. At a second meeting, where guests were chatting around a dinner table, Amis recalled that Powell was paying attention but not contributing much. When he did say something Amis was puzzled by his reference to himself in the third person. But the end was not yet. Amis was making a point when he used the word 'impingement', at which moment, without addressing the subject Amis was discussing, Powell zeroed in pedantically on his use of the word, demanding the etymology. Amis, taken by surprise, tried to explain. 'Alas no, Mr Amis,' said Powell, as he gave him the true derivation, 'I strike a blow,' smacking his fist into his palm for emphasis, making Amis feel, he said, 'a prat'.

At a final meeting Amis spotted Powell standing alone at a party looking baffled. He went up and announced his name. Pursing his lips, Powell said, 'Who?' Amis suggested that most people, if genuinely forgetting a face, would say something like, 'Of course, my dear fellow, how very absurd of me not to have recognised you', especially if they were in politics rather than the 'truth-at-any-price' business. Amis wondered finally what Powell was doing there if parties were so difficult for him.

These descriptions of seemingly rude and certainly baffling social behaviour can be explained when you realise that Enoch Powell was a classic embodiment of Asperger's syndrome.

His lack of political friends and his provocative and frequently self-destructive political behaviour led to Enoch Powell's final sidelining. Like many Aspergers, he was in the wrong job, though he did it as best he could, and sometimes brilliantly, using his supreme intellect to camouflage his gross social ineptitude and lack of political nous. He was probably better suited to the dry world of academe, where, rather than having his name execrated on all sides, as happened after his notorious 1968 Birmingham immigration speech, he would have shone in glory. Or perhaps he would have been happiest teaching young children, with whom he had such a knack; and reading, writing, and thinking in his spare time.

When he died, in 1998, the only Labour politician of significance to attend his funeral was Tony Benn. Despite their diametrically opposed political standpoints, and the instructive differences in the presentation of their autistic traits, these two autonomous politicians shared that essential Asperger's characteristic: a strong, occasionally peculiar, unbendable moral code which led sometimes to professional disaster.

★

Outside Sarah's window, life is going on. I look out at the scudding clouds over the escarpment of the distant Weald, away to the north. On a nearby lamppost a gull is squatting, a crust in its bill. The drain machine is doing its thing, the man in the corner shop is no doubt dressing down his shelves, and the lady in the station café has probably not yet cleaned the congealed brown ketchup from the top of the 1970s plastic-tomato dispenser that I noticed when I walked past earlier.

I've been answering questions and talking about myself for hours. My tea has gone cold. I feel that my answers have been telling a story and, despite the risk of pinning the tail on the wrong bit of the donkey, or even on the wrong donkey, I'm impelled in one direction. This crazy condition, Asperger's syndrome, is making complete sense of the long non sequitur of my sometimes ludicrous, often lonely, and overridingly out-of-sync life.

Sarah puts the top neatly back on her pen and looks across at me.

'Your eye contact today has been unusual,' she says.

'Unusual?'

'Not much of it. Do you want to know what I think?'

'Yes,' I say.

There is a word in the dictionary to describe the kind of physique said to be associated with an introverted, shy, restrained, alert, sensitive, and intellectual temperament. The word is 'cerebrotonic' and the purported body type connected with it is ectomorphic (lean). Sherlock Holmes is of the cerebrotonic type, as am I.

Sarah draws in her breath. 'I think you have Asperger's syndrome,' she says.

I nod in my cerebrotonic way. Somewhere I hear the low pulse of a water pumping station, or is it the throb of the blood in my ears? I feel tremendously at peace.

'How did you work it out exactly?'

'The tests you have done tell me. Our conversation tells me. My experience tells me.'

I nod again.

'Your AQ score is well within the autistic range, and your answers to my questions are also indicative.'

'I'm not arguing,' I say. 'You're only confirming what I'd already decided for myself.'

Sarah smiles, like the Secretary of the Magic Circle having just admitted a new member to the exclusive club.

'Most adults who seek diagnosis are correct in their guess,' she says. 'They've done all the legwork.'

'So,' I say, 'Asperger's syndrome. That explains everything.' Sarah looks at me steadily. The crawling sunbeams have reached the junction of the floor and wall. Motes of dust hang in the still air.

'Is there anything else that gave you a clue?' I ask.

Sarah closes her file slowly and looks at me. 'I need to be careful what I say. This process is standardised, the tests are all well established and properly approved, and I'm punctilious. We take great care to avoid over-assessing, over-diagnosing.'

I nod for a third time.

'Look,' she says, 'I've diagnosed six hundred people, and seen many more over the years. But sometimes you can just tell as soon as somebody walks through the door. You know the term "gaydar", the word gay people have for the instinctive "gay radar" they use to identify other gay people? Well, I use the word "adar". It's radar for autism. You just spot it. I spotted it in several members of my immediate family.'

I'm still trying to get a grip on how Asperger's syndrome fits into the whole autism picture, I tell her.

'Asperger's is part of autism,' explains Sarah. 'The different bit between classic autism and Asperger's syndrome is intellectual capacity. What's the same is the autism.'

'But I know people who have told me they've got Asperger's syndrome,' I say, 'and they seem different to me.'

'When you overlay normal brain scans they all look pretty much the same,' says Sarah. 'When you overlay autistic brains things look different. There's no such thing as a typical person with Asperger's. For example, you have insight into your condition. Not everybody does.'

I can still hear the drain-sucking elephant doing its work further up the street. I wonder what the capacity of the tanker would look like in pictures. How many gallons of drain water? How many pints? How many teacupfuls?

I realise that Sarah is looking at me, expecting an answer to some question.

'Sorry,' I say, 'I got distracted by something — zoned out.'

'It happens,' she says. 'I was asking about your family. Any signs there might be autism anywhere else?'

I stop to think. I have a son in his twenties, Jake, a solitary like me. I always knew I was a law unto myself, and he is the same. Possibly more so. He is a musician, a bright chap, and unusual. I have noticed his intense absorptions since childhood, first skateboarding and computer games, and then, lastingly, music. He spends all day practising. Of course many boys enjoy these things, but perhaps not in so focused and uncompanionable a way. Then there is his obsession with cold showers and cold-water swimming. I have also observed his flat indifference to things in which he is not interested, and his firm disinclination to fit in if he does not want to. He has a couple of good friends but not many, and some are twenty or thirty years older than him. In this he reminds me of myself.

Under a passive stubborn surface he is an anxious and very emotional young fellow. When he was little I used to take him every day to infant school. As we approached he would become silent and withdrawn, and as I tried to hand him over he would cling to me and cry in desperation. He was unusually distressed and it never got better over the years. I was told that once he was there, in the very structured environment, he gradually calmed down. But dropping him off every day was hard. Afterwards, I remember, I used to sit quietly in the car for a minute or two to recover.

'I sometimes wonder about my son,' I say. I mention that Jake's strangeness reminds me, and other people, of my brother Paul, also a musician and also odd in a way that's hard to pin down. Like Paul, Jake is a 'present-dweller' who finds planning hard.

'Keep an eye out,' says Sarah, 'It's very heritable, autism. Runs in families.'

She arranges her things, which I recognise as a signal that the session is coming to a close. I take a draught of water from the glass with the tiny bubbles.

'Well,' says Sarah Hendrickx, rising from her chair, 'I'll email you a complete report next week.'

'I won't shake hands,' I say.

'Of course you won't,' she says, as she sees me out into the street with a smile.

I walk down the road in the spring sunshine. I feel like the man who has finally gone to the doctor because he keeps falling over, and the doctor says, 'But you've only got one leg. Didn't you notice?' I've been falling over socially and in other ways my whole life — at school, with my family, at work, down the pub — but it never occurred to me that there might be some reason for it, something that explained why I was the way I was and that maybe there were other people like me who processed the world rather as I did. Perhaps I wasn't, as I'd thought, mad; perhaps I wasn't, as I'd thought, *alone*. I had unwittingly been autistic, an Asperger, my whole life.

★

A lot of water seems to have flowed under the bridge since I last saw Odette Pinard, but she has suggested a final meeting, to catch up. The room is bright and cheerful as I sit down and I feel rather chipper, as if I have just discovered the lost manuscripts of Johann Sebastian Bach down the back of the sofa. Odette is looking over my anxiety and depression form.

'You seem about as anxious as usual,' she says, 'but you're reporting no depression. A complete change from your previous forms.'

'It's gone,' I say. 'I've been depressed to a greater or lesser degree, I suppose, since about 1973, but since my diagnosis it has lifted entirely. It's very strange. I feel, well, not exactly buoyant, but hopeful. Some days I feel almost normal. For the first time in a long time I'm actually looking forward to tomorrow.'

'Well, zat is good news,' says Odette so exuberantly that her French accent pokes for a moment above the surface. 'Let's hope it continues.'

'It will,' I say, 'I know it.'

Odette puts her chin in her hand and looks at me sideways. 'I don't think there's any need to continue with the rest of this session, do you?'

'No,' I say.

'I think the discovery we've come upon together has made a real difference to you, Tom.'

'It has,' I say as I stand up, wondering exactly how the royalties for this joint discovery should be split.

As Odette sees me out she gives me a warm smile, which I return. There is nothing Pan Am about it this time.

In the waiting room I pass the usual collection of 'frequent-flyers'. On the stairs the sun is striking the jazzy painting, giving it a summery, cheerful appearance. I walk home through the park, where laughing children are at play.

A few days later an email headed 'Autism Spectrum Assessment' arrives from Sarah Hendrickx. The niceties are explained and there is a brief outline of the screening tools. On the Autism Quotient the average person scores about 17. Eighty per cent of those with a diagnosis of Asperger's syndrome score 32 or more. My AQ Score is 37. On the Empathy Quotient typical people score around 45. Eighty per cent of diagnosed Aspergers score 30 or less. My EQ score is 20.

The overall assessment takes into account a spread of other characteristics:

> Tom is a concrete thinker, with difficulties in reading people and social signals, which results in social awkwardness and difficulties in understanding the emotional perspectives of others. He has some lifelong intense interests (including road signs and type). Tom's experiences of anxiety and depression could be related to this atypical cognitive profile and its impact on a sense of 'fitting in'. From the test scores, observation, and information provided Tom could meet the diagnostic criteria for Autism Spectrum Condition (Asperger Syndrome).

Here it is in black and white: 'Tom could meet the diagnostic criteria for Autism Spectrum Condition (Asperger Syndrome)'. I note the use of the self-protective conditional tense and the amusingly mild term 'atypical cognitive profile'. The report is at once commonplace and revelatory. I know in my bones that after more than half a century of fumbling I've got a hat that fits. No longer do I feel neurotic, stupid, or mad. It's all come a bit late. But better late than never.

Now that I understand myself, I can plan. I can explain myself to people. Maybe I'll see a change in their expectations. Perhaps allowances will be made. Perhaps some of my curious behaviour, my confusion and exhaustion in society, will be understood, or at least acknowledged. All the same, I don't want to indulge in unrealistic expectations. I will see how it goes. It has been five-and-a-half decades since the autism fairy landed on my cot and uttered her malediction. It will probably take a bit of time to unpick the threads of her spell. There is so much I want to tell Lea.

I wonder: have I got good autism radar? I think about some of the people I have known and a new light is cast upon a few of them. There was awkward Azif, who flapped his hands when excited. He was an editor at a listings magazine before he left to work on time-tables for a bus company. He wore plastic shoes, was an authority on pub signs, and subscribed to a magazine called *Modern Railways*. I recall a boy at school: handsome, withdrawn, incredibly bright, an expert in many subjects, though very passive. He was regularly set upon by bullies but refused to defend himself, though he was quite big enough. Instead he would quietly take it, emerging at the end dripping blood onto his white school shirt. There is the fantastically anxious Donald, a retired BBC engineer and computer nerd of astonishing pedantry, and clever Linda, strangely dressed,

123

with a masculine haircut and dark hair on her arms. She loves vintage motorcars and talks about them in a monotonous stream. Then there's Gary, the solitary, loping 3D-map maker who looks at the table while he's talking to you and wears bowler hats and frock coats in the street. He is a world-famous juggler, the proprietor of a flea circus, and a superb instrumentalist on anything you care to name from the euphonium to the penny whistle. His father was an engineer. Tiny temple bells are tinkling. These are fellow travellers, in whom I recognise something shared.

I decide to get some fresh air. As I shut the front door the familiar wetland tang drifts up from the salt marshes along the river. I pass through the churchyard, where a wagtail is twitching in the crook of a branch. As the clock chimes four a blackbird launches itself from behind a clump of rosemary, rising in a helix around the tower of the church. A gentle breeze flutters the flowers beside the graves and specks of pollen drift among the sunbeams. I am Tom Cutler. It is an absolutely glorious day.

Chapter 3:
Loose chippings

The child is father of the man

WILLIAM WORDSWORTH

I was born in the maternity wing of a Welsh hospital on a blustery November Thursday in 1959. Food rationing had been over for five years, *Mack The Knife* was topping the charts, and people had never had it so good.

Within weeks of my birth, my dad moved us to Plymouth, a town he knew well. It was the place where he and my mother had met. I was their first child, and if my Welsh birth didn't mark me as an outsider something else did: my parents were Roman Catholics.

My dad was born in London, in 1931, one of three children.

His father was an engineer and was well enough to do, owning a house, and a large black car against which the family posed for photographs. But there was more to this man than met the eye: he was a serial bigamist, who left in his wake a string of baffled wives and children in countries as far flung as England and Australia.

If having a bigamist father was not enough for my dad, there was also something seriously wrong with his mother. This woman cast a sombre shadow, beating her children with a stick, chattering insanely, and writing letters to the Pope. 'She was out of this world,' said my dad, 'quite out of it. I think she was mad, in the old sense of the word.'

One day, when my father was a young boy, my grandfather walked out, unwilling any longer to deal with his profoundly damaged wife. 'Your father's gone,' said his mother, without ceremony. Of course, walking out on a wife and children was his thing, but in going he removed a vital footing from this house of cards. 'When Dad left,' my father told me, 'things went haywire.'

My father's mother being judged incompetent to care for him, he was put into a Catholic boarding school, where he spent the first part of the Second World War. Here he was diagnosed with tuberculosis, then still a killer, and on D-Day, 6 June 1944, as the first paratroopers leapt into the unknown over the high cliffs of 'Omaha' beach, an old surgeon was brought out of retirement to cut the tubercular glands from my father's neck. Afterwards, he was dispatched to convalesce in a hut in the grounds of a Catholic convent. During this time, and though he was just twelve, his mother refused to visit him.

The convent gardener, a kindly and shrewd conscientious objector, recognised in this lost child a soul in grave need of stability and care. He tipped off the staff at Blackfriars School, Laxton, a sort of junior seminary run by the Dominicans, a religious order of preaching friars.

Named after St Dominic, and known as the 'Black Friars' for the dark cape they sometimes wear over their habit, the Dominicans took my father under their wing, feeding, accommodating, and indoctrinating him, with a mixture of practical charity, Dominican intellectualism, and boarding-school rice pudding, to which, along with cricket, rugby, and the austere Latin liturgy, he retains an attachment to this day. The Dominicans not only sheltered my father from his disordered mother, but for six years they really looked after him.

In his time at Laxton, my dad was being prepared for the priesthood and on leaving school he spent a probationary year as a novice friar at Woodchester Priory in Stroud before moving to Hawkesyard Priory in Staffordshire for a further three years' study. In family albums from this time there are snaps of him in his white habit, looking like a young Gregory Peck in a film about the Ku Klux Klan.

My father was nonplussed by some of the men attracted to the religious life. They included a chap who, as he lowered a coffin into a grave, forgot to feed the webbing through his hands and ended on his stomach with his arms stretched down into the hole, and another who, he said, used to fart under his habit, whispering, 'It stinks worse than Jerusalem.' These peculiar events, though seldom mentioned at the dinner table, supplied the soft background music to my growing up.

Since the thirteenth century, the Dominicans had operated a religious community and theological study centre as part of Oxford University. And so it was to Blackfriars Oxford that my father went for the final stretch of his bookwormish journey to the priesthood.

But in the end he did not become a priest, leaving Blackfriars in the spring of 1956, after only eight months. 'I couldn't stand it!' he told me, 'I didn't know what I wanted to do.' He had been seen as a safe pair of hands, a Dominican mover and shaker of the future, so when, after all those years of Greek, Latin, and hard theological graft, he dropped the bombshell, his mentors at Blackfriars were surprised and possibly hurt. 'We thought you were one of the blessed,' they told him. But, understanding and kind, they kitted him out with clothes, money, and their best wishes, and sent him on his way, out into the real world.

It was going to be quite a cold bath.

★

My father had a friend, Ralph, from his days at Laxton. Ralph was living in Plymouth with his new wife Kit, and knowing my dad's need for a roof over his head, they invited him to live with them.

One day, Kit's darkly attractive sister, Sarah, came to dinner. She had a flat on the Hoe, where Sir Francis Drake is supposed to have played a game of bowls before seeing off the Spanish Armada in 1588. No longer bound by vows of poverty, chastity, and obedience, my father made his move.

But there was a complication. In 1956, conscription still had four years to run and my dad was required to do two years of National Service. The Cold War was hotting up and, along with a handpicked bunch of other oddballs, some of them heading for British spy organisations, my father was selected to learn Russian. It may be that his close-mouthed, solitary, studious character identified him as good spy material. In any case, he was sent to the remote Joint Services School for Linguists in Crail, a cobbled fishing village on the east coast of Scotland.

The JSSL course was notoriously tough, involving day after day of gruelling instruction from a jumble of eccentric Soviet defectors and White Russian émigrés. With the rudiments of Greek and Latin already under his belt, my father spent his days conjugating Russian verbs and memorising lengthy lists of vocabulary. He did this for an impressive five months, but his mind was elsewhere. The trouble was that Crail on the windswept Scottish coast was much too far from Sarah's Plymouth flat.

★

My mother was born in Woolwich, the youngest of six daughters. One afternoon during the war, a German bomb meant for the nearby Royal Arsenal exploded in her street in Bexleyheath. It was a hot day and she recalled coming into the dining room in her knitted bathing costume, where the table had been laid for tea. There was a huge noise and everything went black. As the dust cleared the sunlight revealed the transmogrified tea table, covered in glass. Through the broken window my mother could see planes flying up the River Thames.

The family moved to Harrow on the Hill, on the opposite side of London. Here, they became members of the Catholic parish of Our Lady and St Thomas of Canterbury, where the priest was Father John Hitchcock, a cousin of the aforementioned Alfred Hitchcock. My mother got to know Fr John well. He was a frequent guest at the family home, where her father fed him Scotch whisky while he talked, rapid-fire, about locomotives.

'He was a real train nut,' said my mum.

I pricked up my ears.

'Timetables, tinkering, or trainspotting?' I asked.

'Oh, all of it,' she said, 'He was always on the platform or the footplate. He just loved trains.'

In all my reading about Alfred Hitchcock I have never noticed anything more than a glancing reference to Fr John, and I had certainly never heard of a mania for trains. But knowing what I did about Hitch it immediately struck me as suggestive that his cousin should be a railway 'anorak'. It was fascinating to learn in this personal way that in at least two members of the Hitchcock family there were signs of Asperger's syndrome.

Not long after the end of the war, at the age of just fifty-two, my mother's father took ill and died and my widowed grandmother moved her girls to Pimlico, close to Westminster Cathedral, the Catholic Mother Church.

To me, Grandma seemed the eternal widow, in true Victorian style. A huge black-and-white portrait photograph of her late husband hung on her wall until she died, well into her nineties. She used to say things like 'God bless' and 'It's five-and-twenty past six', and she told me when I was little that there had been no aeroplanes when she was a girl, a story that seemed incredible. I wish I had been able to know her better, but I found her at once standoffish and silly. She was an intelligent woman, but I think her deep anxiety caused her to miss out on a lot of life. Her idea of a good time was reading the Catholic newspaper *The Universe* over a Vesta dehydrated curry.

After my father's demob in 1958, my parents were married by a friend who was a priest. Because my mother was the sister of the wife of my father's friend Ralph, Ralph became one of my future uncles; his wife Kit one of my future aunts; and her sister Sarah my mother-to-be. It was like a music hall song.

Though they had paid for a wedding photographer, my parents decided it was going to cost too much to have the pictures developed, so I have never seen them. Money was tight and my intellectually minded father decided to train as a teacher. In this he was following in the steps of my mother, who had gone into teaching as soon as she finished school.

In the early days, my father taught in a private school in the Cotswolds, where Walter Rothschild had once ridden around in a carriage drawn by zebras. Here, he told me with obvious regret, and possibly recalling his own childhood, he used to beat disobedient pupils with a stick. On one occasion he ordered a naughty boy to stand on his chair.

'Hands in the air!' he demanded.

'But, Sir, I've got a withered arm,' explained the boy.

'Then put your leg in the air!' barked my father.

Though he can sometimes appear fierce, my dad is actually an enormously kind and thoughtful man who had every skill needed for teaching and caring for primary-school children, at which he became expert.

Like Enoch Powell and Alfred Hitchcock, he has a knack for children, which you might not guess from his demeanour in the library, where he spends so much of his time. He was greatly loved by those he taught, and this was partly because of his eccentric methods, such as stomping across the class on top of the children's desks.

One weekend, years ago, he took me into his empty school, a place of varnish and echoes. At the front of his classroom, a child's desk had been connected to his own by several strands of wool, carefully taped there by the troubled little girl whose seat it was. 'What do you think that means?' he asked, lifting a rhetorical eyebrow.

Good though he is with youngsters, my father has never been quite so adept with adults. He managed the formalities of parents' evenings perfectly well, but ordering in a pub or talking to a trades-man or to neighbours he is, like my mother to a lesser degree, ill at ease, and does not seem quite sure how to relate to other human beings. I used to put this down to his cloistered upbringing, but I have recently come to the conclusion that his strange social behaviour is a sign that he shares with me more than a scintilla of Asperger's syndrome.

It is common for the parents of children with Asperger's to display signs of it themselves. Sometimes these signs are frank but often they are subtle. In the case of my own father there are several tantalising clues to the possibility that my autism springs from family DNA, though these can fade like ghosts if you turn the light on them.

My dad has a number of 'special interests'. The trouble is that these may not be autistic; they might be ordinary human enthu-siasms. Since his retirement many years ago, he has, for example, made a deep study of international jurisprudence. But this could just be an uncommonly intellectual hobby. Perhaps the most intri-guing of his enthusiasms is the one he has for a certain brand of weatherproof clothing, which he sometimes wears indoors, and which he will tell you about in great detail at the slightest provoca-tion. This is certainly an offbeat interest, but has it crossed the line into autistic perseveration?

My father's dress sense is somewhat whimsical, veering towards the nerdish. He can look perfectly smart in a conventional lounge suit or Harris Tweed jacket, and tie, but his trousers and shoes often appear ungainly and strangely matched. At home, unlike anyone else I have seen, he habitually wears his shirt collars unturned-down, the points poking upwards into his chin.

Like me, my father does not like to be touched. He will

surrender to a handshake but will not initiate one, and seated next to another person he looks uneasy. Of course, this may just be his English reserve or his austere upbringing, but I have a feeling that he shares with me the Asperger's 'keep clear gene'. He is not a hugger. Watching him say goodbye to some visitors recently, I took care to observe his behaviour. First, he stood up, rigidly, with a confused smile on his face. People were leaving and it was clear to him that he was expected to react. As his daughter-in-law embraced him he attempted to reciprocate, but it was an action involving the arms only, he remained stiff as a tree. He circled her waist but kept his fists closed, bumping his knuckles rhythmically against her back.

When saying goodbye, I myself go through a repertoire of uncomfortable movements similar to my dad's, which make me look and feel gauche. Many have remarked on it, and it is only with children, and with very affirmative or vigorous people who override my apparently disdainful spasticity and just grab hold of me, that I relax slightly and can return the embrace in a more normal way.

Being essentially a formal, non-social, and non-reciprocal enterprise, teaching was an ideal job for my dad, as it often is for those with Asperger's. The absent-minded professor, a classic Asperger's caricature, is in his or her element in the one-way environment of the classroom or university lecture hall.

★

Between 1959 and 1966 my parents produced a new child nearly every year. Several of us were touched in our cradle by the finger of autism, but it left its print more sharply on some than on others. Until my diagnosis, I'm sure the idea of autism in the immediate family had never occurred to my parents, or to my siblings. Apart from me, none of us has had a formal assessment or diagnosis. Perhaps now they might.

As the first child, I had the undivided attention of my mother until the birth of my sister Esther, at home, twenty months later. I was naturally resentful of the impostor, who, as she got older, seemed increasingly haughty. Though Esther could laugh and smile as well as anyone, she could also look disapproving. Even today she retains the forbidding habit of clasping her arms unsmilingly around herself as you talk, watching you expressionless like an eagle owl ready to strike. At times, she can appear injudicious or tactless in her comments, seeming to scoff. But this is not her intention and never has been, because, of course, Esther is exhibiting her personal variety of my own Aspergic critical severity, and, as with my own apparent aloofness, any offence is unintended.

Esther's all-engulfing interest is in music making, and she is a superb teacher of music to children. She will enlarge on her subject at length, with enthusiasm, expertise, and great warmth, with whatever personal news you might bring into the conversation being quickly swept along by the rushing musical tide.

In 1961, we were living above a working-men's club in Plymouth and my parents, who were both teaching, were looking for someone to take care of me and Esther during the day. Opposite us were some post-war prefabs and it was in one of these that they found a lady called Mary, whose two sons were growing up and who missed having young children around. I took to Mary and her quiet good sense at once, christening her 'Auntie'. When my baby sister stuck a doll's eye up her nose and my parents were not sure what to do Mary administered pepper. Simple, effective, and loud.

Auntie Mary was married to David, a jeweller, and in due

course they became my godparents. Auntie told my mother that I insisted on them endlessly marching with me round the coffee table. It was little surprise when a bemused neighbour, unable to see me below the level of the window, asked Auntie why she and her respectable husband incessantly circled their sitting room like prisoners on exercise.

I had a persistent interest in Auntie's oven door, which I would open and close repeatedly. I also liked to wrap myself very tightly in the curtain and then spin round and round as it unwound. Was this interest in the oven door, this circling and spinning, normal childish behaviour or was something else going on here?

My language acquisition was going according to expectations and Auntie took me on trips to the library. In this hushed temple of learning, her two sons encouraged me to shout 'bugger'. We were sent outside, where they made me shout 'bugger' louder, through the letter flap. Auntie took it well.

I always liked strong flavours and still do: fermented Baltic herring, horseradish, smoky Scotch whisky with a smack of the medicine cabinet. The first taste I remember is liquorice. My mother was standing by a sunny window eating a stick of something dark and aromatic. Bending down from her immense height she handed me a tiny piece of the black stuff. As I tried it I looked up at her and asked how old she was. Thirty she said. This seemed tremendously ancient. I must have been about three.

Though very shy and anxiety-prone, I was an inquisitive child. One day my pet tortoise died and I have never forgotten the solemn ceremony of interment, led by my father in the back garden. Life was full of new things.

Sometimes 'Uncle' David would show me magic tricks. I remember sitting in his musty shed, the rain drumming on the corrugated roof as he passed a coin magically through the table. From that moment, magic became my intense preoccupation. I tried to imitate the tricks I saw but without success. The simple mechanics hadn't occurred to me. I never lost this enthusiasm, and as a teenager I used to sit alone for hours in my bedroom, practising, practising. Whenever I perform today I try to produce in my audience that same feeling of wonder at seeing *real magic*, which I felt so powerfully as a little boy.

But my father's life was still darkened by the baleful penumbra of my impossible grandmother, who, though now in a distant town, would make unannounced visits. My dad told me that as a child he had once squirted her with a water pistol and that she had turned on him. So he let her have it with both barrels, at which she completely collapsed. 'I learnt that this was how I had to treat her,' he said. When sent to fetch the silver-topped cane with which she intended to beat him he began to refuse, instead hiding under the table, where she was unable to reach him because of her girth. Now, though, she was wilder, weirder, and more unhinged than ever. My father decided that to protect his growing family and save his own mental health decisive action was needed: he must do something drastic to escape his mother's destructive sway.

One dark night I was woken and put into my dressing gown, my baby sister Esther was bundled up, and my dad closed the front door. I am often at a loss to know why people are behaving as they are, though I have always been highly sensitive to mood. Even at the age of three, the hushed voices and urgent whispers told me that something momentous was afoot, though I didn't know what.

Auntie was there in the darkness. In her strong Devon accent, she whispered that Mum and Dad and Esther and I were going away. She had made a tray of toffee for me to take with me. I looked down at the golden squares, separated by strips of greaseproof paper. I didn't want to leave Auntie. I loved her. It was all very mysterious.

We were driven to a railway station and my parents squeezed the four of us into a sleeping car. Brisk goodbyes were exchanged in the dark and the train pulled out. Auntie was waving from the platform, the tray of toffee still in her hand. I sometimes think wistfully of that un-given present.

My father had prepared carefully, telling not even his brother and sister of his intended departure, and erasing from the record all evidence of our new location. Only one or two friends were in the know and they had been briefed to keep quiet. It would be decades before my father's siblings could track him down; he never spoke to his mother again; she ended her days in the locked ward of a Scottish lunatic asylum.

★

We spent the next three years in a leafy Hertfordshire town, where my father had got himself another teaching job. I learnt to swing conkers, and made friends with a girl who came to play in our back garden. She told me that her father's birthday was the same as mine. I argued that this was impossible, as he was much older than me. How confusing the world seemed.

In the afternoons Dad would arrive home from work and post chocolates through the front door, before going round to the kitchen to be greeted by my mother as I investigated the contents of the crumpled paper bag. Mum peeled apples, letting the long spiral of skin fall to the floor. At bedtime she used to sing me to sleep. She had an excellent voice and enjoyed the folk songs made popular by Kathleen Ferrier: 'Blow the Wind Southerly' was a favourite.

Then there was a ditty in French, 'Dominique', an unlikely top-ten hit about St Dominic, written and performed by the 'Singing Nun'. Whenever I hear the song today, I am swept back to my childhood, tucked up tightly in bed, with my mother singing me softly to sleep.

I always wanted heavy blankets on top of me, and still do. A light covering feels unpleasant, like a wind blowing over rustling leaves. This is not an uncommon foible among people with Asperger's syndrome, and when my father recently came to visit he too asked for heavier blankets. I remember reading that the poet W. H. Auden felt the same way. He piled blankets, curtains, and, once, a weighty stair-carpet on top of himself, and slept under those. On another occasion he went to bed underneath a heavy oil-painting.

This reminded me of Temple Grandin, one of the best-known autistic speakers in the USA. Grandin is a professor of animal science at Colorado State University and a livestock industry consultant with an eerie understanding of the way cattle think and behave. As a student, she noticed that the simple machine used to hold the animals motionless had a very calming effect on them, so she tried it on herself, with success. She then built her own prototype 'hug box', a version of which is now available for autistic people to use.

W. H. Auden displayed plenty of other features of Asperger's. He had a gawky gait, collected hats, dressed strangely — wearing carpet slippers in public — and spoke in a rather monotonous voice somewhat reminiscent of Alfred Hitchcock's. A year before his death, he appeared on BBC Television's *Parkinson* show revealing several giveaway Asperger traits, the most immediately obvious being his marked lack of eye contact with the interviewer.

In 1964, my mother produced a second son, Paul, my only brother. Paul was a bright boy, but as he grew up he became known for his peculiar ways. When tired or excited he would rock rhythmically backwards and forwards. 'Why does your brother do that?' people would ask. I didn't know. Nobody asked why I touched various 'significant' lampposts on my way to school, jiggled my teeth compulsively from side to side, or bounced my legs rhythmically under the desk. They didn't ask because I did it discreetly, as I still do.

Though we didn't know it, Paul's rocking and, I now believe, my own jittering and object touching, were examples of autistic 'stimming'.

In time Paul's rocking faded, as did his charming naivety, and he developed the ability to tell disablingly funny stories about his own frequent mishaps. He is truly terrible at following directions. Pointing him towards my local station once, I told him: 'Go up to the end of the road and turn left', patting his left arm for emphasis. I watched him walk up to the junction and look around abstractedly, before turning *right*.

We were all therefore astonished when, at the age of about thirteen, and long before the days of smartphone maps, Paul took the train to London, found his way to Sotheby's, and nonchalantly joined in an auction of antique lutes.

He learnt to read music with no difficulty but found the reading of words and sentences onerous. My mother spent so long trying to show him the difference between 'bed' and 'deb' that she briefly made remedial teaching her speciality. Today, Paul is a talented musician and teacher, with a wife and grown-up children, but he is still likely to write 'deb' when he means 'bed'.

You did not hear the word 'dyslexia' much in the 1960s and it wasn't until the late 1970s that it started to become clear what was going on in my brother's brain. Dyslexia, or 'word blindness', was first identified in Germany in the 1870s. It is a learning difficulty unrelated to intellectual ability, which chiefly affects reading, writing, and language. Like Asperger's syndrome, it is commonly associated with quirks of short-term memory, slow processing speed, poor organisation and sequencing, and unusual time perception. Dyslexics seem to have a problem with a bit of chromosome 7 known as 7q31, an area that has also been linked to autism, and it is common for autism and dyslexia to be present in the same person, as they are in my brother.

Like Aspergers, dyslexics are often bright and articulate, though they may do badly at school. They frequently share Aspergers' difficulty in maintaining attention and can 'zone out', daydream, and lose track of time. Uninformed and unimaginative teachers will see them as careless, immature, idle, insolent, uncooperative, or several of these. In many of these ways my brother and I are alike. The main difference is that he has trouble with written words and I have a facility with them.

★

One afternoon, when I was about five, I was standing at the kitchen door, looking into our Hertfordshire garden and preparing to take off my boots. My mother was playing with Esther and Paul, who were sitting in a tin pedal-car. My dad was at work. Ready to pull off the first boot, I braced myself against the doorjambs when all at once the wind slammed the door on my fingers. I next remember hanging over my mum's shoulder, pouring blood down her white cardigan as she tried to decide what to do with me. We had no car and no telephone. Somehow she raised a neighbour.

We were driven to the hospital while the neighbour's wife looked after my brother and sister. As a nurse removed the homemade bandage I could see that the top of the middle finger of my left hand was hanging off, attached by a flap of flesh. The bone had been narrowly missed so they gave me a local anaesthetic and sewed the hinge back on. Most of this time I was making loud noises of one sort or another.

I was bandaged up and taken to a sweetshop where my mother said I could choose anything I wanted. I went for a chocolate rabbit wrapped in brightly coloured foil. I had never been presented with such an enormous sweet. It looked about a foot high. I tried to peel back the foil but my injured finger, encased in a leather fingerstall, was in the way. When I finally bit into the chocolate I was dismayed to find it a hollow shell. The disappointment was huge, and the cynical deception of the manufacturers still bothers me today. This might seem an ungrateful overreaction, especially after all this time, but I now understand my sensitivity to this deceit as a typical facet of my Asperger self. The insight, a recent one, is a great relief, for to understand is to forgive.

When they cut the bandages off a few weeks later, the pale digit that emerged had an impressive scar running around its top. To this day, the end of this finger is slightly misshapen. Noticing it once, a friend said, 'I've always wanted something like that.'

★

One Christmas morning, my father called me into my mother's bedroom.

'Come and look at this,' he said.

I peered into the cot at the end of the bed.

'Is it a baby?' I asked.

'Yes, she's your new sister, Rebecca.'

There were now four of us: me, Esther, Paul, and Rebecca.

Having your birthday on Christmas Day seemed like bad luck, and maybe it was, as Rebecca's trademark, like my mother's, would turn out to be anxiety. Growing up, she would sometimes be overcome by sudden terrors, calling out 'I don't want to die. I don't want to be nothing' before dissolving into tears. On one such alarming occasion in the car, my father said to her, 'Remember, you were nothing once … and for a long time.'

All this child production meant that my mother was either pregnant and working, or taking months off to nurse the latest infant, before starting the game all over again. With her hands full, it fell to my father to walk me to my infant school.

One day we found ourselves approaching a dustcart. These things have always repelled me. I notice the reek of rotting rubbish long before anyone else. It's the same in the supermarket, where the strongly unpleasant smell of hot bread hits you the minute you walk in — I'm told other people like it — and the powerful plastic odour of the electrical department and the stench of the fish counter are eye-watering. People say I make too much of smells, but I am very alert to them. They disturb me.

As we passed the dustcart I must have made a face because two brisk nuns walking by remarked on it. They were coming from the school, where on my first day I had been so overcome with anxiety that I was shaking with tears all morning. At playtime I had been approached by one of those people who is in exactly the right job. She was, I suppose, a sort of classroom assistant, and I recall her warm pink cardigan and her blonde hair. She bent down, took my hand, and led me over to join some huge-looking boys who were playing a game. Though I wanted to join in I was dumb with fear.

Back in the class, the uniformed nun who was teaching me told me to stop pulling the woollen bobbles off my jumper. 'Only babies do that,' she said, making a shape with her mouth that resembled the picture of an inflamed anus I once saw in *Nursing Mirror*. Though the word 'logic' was unknown to me, I knew at once that she had made a mistake; her proposition was impossible. A) Being five, I was not a baby, B) I was pulling bobbles off my jumper, therefore, C) It was false that only babies pulled bobbles off their jumpers.

I was the only one of us children to be schooled by nuns, and though I recall the echoes and perfumes of the church, Christian metaphysics baffled me then as it does today. I love the language and crisp carpentry of the King James Bible, but the notion that the universe was constructed by a benevolent omnipotent deity who allows cats to torture mice and whose son was the supernatural offspring of a virgin impregnated by a ghost, is, in the first part, logically incongruous and, in the second, frankly unpersuasive. This story, concocted by tribesmen who didn't know that everything is made of atoms, doubtless helped give meaning to the ups and downs of their lives, as it still does for many today. But now that we are all better informed we should stop teaching children too young to defend themselves that this metaphorical tale is a historical fact like the French Revolution.

Today, the churchgoing in my immediate family has faded away, and quite what my father believes I have not asked, but like me he seems to hold in some regard the poetry and rigour of the Tridentine rite. However, neither he, nor my mother, nor any of us children belongs to any religious group.

Catherine Caldwell-Harris, a psychology professor at Boston University, has found that a person with Asperger's syndrome is twice as likely as a typical member of the population to tick the atheist or agnostic box. One reason, presumably, is that Aspergers, who are already less socially conformist than others, may also find the 'warm and fuzzy' social aspects of church not just unrewarding but positively repugnant. There is also the principle that in order to decide whether or not something is likely to be true you've got to look at the evidence. Compared with more typical people, Aspergers will be less inclined to embrace the notion of 'faith', which is a euphemism for the belief in something for which there is scant evidence. 'Cold' and 'unemotional' it may sound, but another word for it is 'rational'.

★

In 1966, my father got a better job and we moved again, this time to the suburban outskirts of one of the New Towns carefully planned after the war as places to relocate bombed-out Londoners and other 'overspill'. Halfway between London and Brighton, this town had been socially engineered in neighbourhoods, where media lawyers, famous actors, and airline executives lived cheek by jowl with Cockney dinner-ladies and television repairmen. The churches and pubs of the better off tended to be a lot older, and their houses nicer, but nearly everybody's children went to the same schools.

Our family of six moved into a small terraced house opposite a willow-girt millpond. Lying between our front garden and the unfenced water was a large green where we could safely play.

One of the sounds I remember was the regular wail of a siren, which mooed across the neighbourhood like a distant vacuum cleaner whenever a fire engine was on its way to a shout. My mother explained that this was a wartime air raid alert being put to use. After a year or two the sound was heard no more.

Phillip Stone, an older boy, struck up a kind of friendship with me. He showed me where toads and grass snakes lived and once handed me a slowworm, smooth as gravy. He taught me to identify butterflies in the fields around us, and as I grew older I began to net them myself, systematically pinning them to boards, like Stapleton the naturalist in *The Hound of the Baskervilles*, with their proper Latin names in my best handwriting underneath.

Phillip was what was known as a 'rough boy' but he was a survivor. He could pee amazingly high against the railway bridge that took commuters to London and he really understood how the world worked, in a way I never will. Phillip's worldliness complemented my fastidiousness, and when I was six or seven he gave me my first sex education lesson, behind the garages, using nothing more than a stick and a bottle.

Our house turned out to be too small and we moved into a bigger one, which made national headlines forty years later when a man living there was found guilty of conspiring to cause explosions. It is weird to see on the news the gate through which you used to pass day after day being sealed with police tape, and to imagine people plotting to blow up the Bluewater shopping centre in the room where you once did your English homework.

Soon after we moved in, a girl who lived nearby and always seemed to have mud on her face showed me how to cook potatoes on a campfire that she built in a neighbouring copse. Afterwards she hitched up her dress and weed into the ashes. Fascinating.

One day, a huge Alsatian dog chased me across that copse, knocking me down and biting my elbow. Dogs, like people, have an uncanny knack of picking up on the alert discomfiture I think I hide so well, and it can make them aggressive. I have been wary of dogs ever since, which doesn't help.

I became interested in the wild mushrooms that grew

abundantly in the copse, like the shaggy ink cap, or 'lawyer's wig', which you could eat, but which would turn into a black puddle if you left it on your table overnight. I got a mushroom book out of the library and inspected the family tree. It was rewarding to discover, list, classify, and systemise the various fungi; I was especially allured by the poisonous ones, such as the destroying angel, a tall white phallus of death.

Before long, my sister Ruth was born. Being the youngest, she was allowed a lot more freedom, and received a more dilute dose of the ambient family anxiety. I used to think it was this that had made her the most socially sophisticated of us, but I now believe it was merely the fall of the genetic dice that had allowed her to dodge the autistic finger.

Because the half-curse half-gift of our Aspergic autism was not then recognised for what it was, we tended to be regarded by others as 'odd'. And we still are. At a recent birthday party, Ruth told me: 'Only two people described our family as "strange" tonight. That's a good score.'

Despite their own unusualness, my parents made friends in the New Town. There was a man with a beard who decades later would have something to do with the headline grabbing 'literacy hour', and another man, about seven-feet tall, who was News Editor of the BBC World Service at Bush House. When you saw him and his very tiny wife together they appeared to be members of two distinct species. I also remember a famous scientist who wrote programmes for television, and a solicitor who wore jeans and gave advice about neighbourhood disagreements on the Jimmy Young show. I was impressed by these scintillating with-it people, some of whom had bidets in their bathrooms, or went to bed with women who were not their wives.

Though we had no fridge, telephone, car, or central heating, my parents had aspirations for us. There was a little piano in what we called the back room, and as we got older we were given private music lessons. But with five children under the age of six, and bringing in a modest teacher's salary, my father realised he was going to be bankrupted. It was at this moment that reason overtook the Catholic imperative to multiply, and my parents stopped producing offspring.

My new junior school was a jangle of loud noises and strong odours. The days were punctuated by bells, slamming doors, a racket of voices down echoing corridors, the squeak of chalk on blackboard, and the rebarbative pong of school dinners. These incessant demands on my senses produced in me a condition of highly alert threat readiness, and low-grade anxiety. I was said to be a 'sensitive' boy.

To be absorbed in something was a relief. I was fascinated by patterns and spent hours at my desk with a pair of compasses painstakingly drawing circles and superimposing arcs that generated a multitude of new, segmented shapes, which I would systematically colour. I produced a great many of these motifs and became engrossed while I was making them. With commendable understatement my teacher noted in a school report: 'Thomas seems very taken with work of this kind.'

Somewhere in his past, my father had learned the craft of bookbinding. One day, he showed me how to cut the boards to size and how to make the spine using a special tough paper. He taught me to mitre the corners, attach the end papers, and stick the whole thing together with paste. Finally, he handed me a thin celluloid stencil punched with an alphabet of capital letters, along with a stiff shorthaired brush and a red pigment block. With these tools you could put a title on your book.

My dad told me that the typeface was Monotype Gill Sans and that it had been designed by the Catholic sculptor, stonecutter, and printmaker Eric Gill. I fell in love with the process and spent so many hours, days, weeks, and months using the stencil that, without realising what was happening, I absorbed into myself the anatomy of the fifty-two letterforms and their punctuation marks.

This happy accident opened the door to the world of typography, a world governed by system, formality, detail, and rules. You knew where you were.

I used my pocket money to buy sheets of rubdown letters, which were a bit sticky on the back so that by laying the translucent sheet over a piece of paper marked up with your faint pencil guidelines you could rub down the letters and make words. I learnt the names of these typefaces: Helvetica, Univers, Bembo, Garamond, Baskerville, and got to know their strengths and foibles. I made a thousand mistakes, which is the way you learn.

Whether it was the letters themselves or the deeply satisfying diagrammatic unity that first attracted me to British road signs I cannot recall. Neither do I remember when I became aware of their systematic rigour and beauty; it was probably some time in the early 1970s, though it was not till years later that I learnt how these signs came to look the way they do.

One day in the mid-1950s, a designer named Jock Kinneir was waiting at a bus stop when he got into conversation with a fellow passenger. This man was David Alford, an architect working on the huge expansion of Gatwick Airport. Alford liked the cut of Kinneir's jib and without more ado offered him a hundred guineas to design the airport's signage system.

As his assistant Kinneir hired Margaret Calvert, one of his students at Chelsea Art School, where he taught. Calvert remembers that she had to look up 'typography' in the dictionary. But the pair produced a pioneering signage system in yellow and black.

In 1957, the government decided that special signage was needed for Britain's new motorway network and asked Kinneir and Calvert to come up with a scheme of signs that could be understood in all weathers at decision-making distance by drivers going at speed.

The pair decided to go back to square one. Their focus would be on crystal clear diagrammatic rigour, supreme legibility under the special conditions obtaining on motorways, and, importantly, attractive appearance.

They decided that the signs needed a new set of typographic characters. They wanted a type design of cardinal unambiguity, but one that would, 'sit well in the English landscape'. Kinneir and Calvert based their new type family on a scrupulously clean nineteenth-century sans-serif design. For absolute clarity they adapted specific letter shapes, producing conspicuous differences in otherwise similar characters, such as the curve at the foot of the lower-case l, 'borrowed' from Edward Johnston's brilliant 1916 London Underground typeface, which instantly marks out the l as neither a capital I nor the figure 1. They designed oblique fractions without a dividing bar and cut aslant the strokes of several letters, so helping to retain the word shape of place names. These had had to be widely letterspaced so as to counteract the effect of 'halation' caused by the glare of reflected headlights. As an aid to mass production they put each character onto its own uniquely proportioned 'invisible' tile, so that words could be perfectly spaced by non-specialists. Their new type, soon named Transport, was a great success in tests.

Kinneir came up with a profoundly simple layout structure for the new signs, based on the width of the capital letter I, which

Margaret Calvert rightly called 'brilliant'. Under this rigid rule-governed system, motorway signs could be newly made at any size while automatically remaining in proportion, as well harmonious and clear.

These pioneering efforts worked brilliantly, and Kinneir and Calvert were soon asked to redesign the signs for all British roads, with Margaret Calvert devising a charming suite of simple pictograms, including the now very well-known 'men at work', 'children', and 'farm animals', the last of which shows the silhouette of a real cow she had known as a girl. For signs such as 'wild horses' and 'wild animals', which featured creatures in motion, she went to the work of the Victorian photographer Eadweard Muybridge, famous for his photographic studies of movement.

Kinneir and Calvert's masterly and beautiful system came into effect on 1 January 1965. It is interesting to think that had it not been for a serendipitous meeting of two men at a bus stop a decade earlier, British road signs would now look quite different, and probably worse.

★

At junior school I met a boy called Jon. Like me, he was good at drawing. We liked to spend our time walking round the playground discussing the geometry of perspective or classifying the dinosaurs. Jon was brainier than me and seemed to forget nothing. When I was seven or eight he introduced me to the work of Picasso, and by the time we were ten he had taught me a good deal about the history of art.

Jon's father, an engineer, was taciturn but focused. Ranged along his mantelpiece were the cups he had won for bowling. His mother was good at crosswords and was surprised one day when she learnt that I had been eating the petals from the roses in her front garden. Hearing recently that the autistic TV naturalist Chris Packham had eaten tadpoles I am unsurprised by my behaviour. Jon told his mother that I insisted on sticking stamps onto envelopes upside-down and she maintained that I must be an anarchist.

Jon and I were cast in a school play about the Flood. Jon got the part of God and I got Mrs Noah. It seemed a mirror of real life. In fact, the casting was inspired. Mrs Gossop, our first primary-school teacher, wrote in my school report, 'Thomas is going through what I can only describe as a silly phase.' I have yet to grow out of it. Like many Aspergers, I enjoy silliness of all kinds and being a grotesque suited me. I am always relaxed when showing off on stage: finally alone and in control, anxiety drains away.

Jon's older brother was also intensely bright. He spoke in an odd staccato, was tremendously good at maths, and had various absorbing interests, including horror films, on which subject he must have been some sort of world expert. He went on to study maths at Cambridge University.

Jon himself was and is a walking encyclopaedia. In a bookshop with me recently he picked up a jazz dictionary. 'Several mistakes in this,' he said. 'Here — Wes Montgomery's brother was born on the *thirtieth* of January 1930, not the thirteenth.' He has remained my greatest friend for fifty years and people sometimes ask if we are brothers.

Every fifth of November, the best firework display in town was put on by the Cornfoots, who lived across the road. The perpetually grinning Mr Cornfoot wore a cap made of some coconut-matting type of material, and over his vast brown belly a short gravy-stained vest. Every third tooth was chipped or missing and his wife looked like the Bird Woman from *Mary Poppins*. The Cornfoots' front garden was full of the earliest forms of supermarket trolley, and their children, ranging in age from six months to about forty years, were forever tinkering with vans.

On bonfire night, the Cornfoots' fireworks brought observers in their Minis and Morris Minors from far afield. Starting with half a dozen white-streak rockets, the display built over hours until its phenomenal climax turned the sky orange, like an accident in an armaments factory. In the morning, my brother and I would wander the neighbourhood collecting the eggy-smelling bodies of the dead Sky Hunters.

Our own bonfire night was different, safety being the main concern. The handful of inexpensive fireworks were kept in a biscuit tin, as recommended in alarming public information films on the television, and my father would jump up and down if anybody went near them. Like a bomb disposal man, it took him ten minutes to approach an extinguished Roman candle in case it came to life again, and he would retreat from a lit rocket like a sprinter, pushing us all up against the house. The whole anxiety-ridden performance lasted hours, even though there were only a dozen anorexic fireworks, and we were all grateful to get in again, warm our frozen fingers around the gas fire, and watch the culmination of the Cornfoots' extravaganza, with a mug of cocoa.

I had always wanted to play the banjo and was a fan of a man named Earl Scruggs, who I heard playing the theme tune to a television show called *The Beverly Hillbillies*. One day my father came home with a nylon-strung guitar, which seemed like a related thing, so I asked for lessons.

I was taught a fingerpicking style in which the right thumb plays an alternating one–two on the bass strings while the fingers of the same hand pick out the melody. I remember the feeling of triumph the day I mastered the technique, which enabled me to tackle Elizabeth Cotten's *Freight Train*, a tune I play to this day. Fingerpicking became my new enthusiasm and for the next three years every spare minute was spent practising away in the corner. But I couldn't join a band. I was always a soloist. It was a case again of *other people*.

Our junior school teacher Mr Sturn had been a prisoner of the Japanese and showed us how to clean our teeth without toothpaste. He said things like 'rattling good yarn' and 'ruddy nuisance', and encouraged Jon and me in our studies of modern art, though he disliked Picasso and found Cézanne 'too plain', preferring soft-focus pink flowers in a nice frame. I looked down my nose at his taste in a priggish, unpleasant way.

It was soon time to move up to the local senior school, which had been a grammar but which, by absorbing the next-door secondary modern, had recently become a comprehensive. The whip-like deputy-head, who played the bassoon and wore a gown during assemblies, was dismayed by the influx into his school of secondary modern boys, and now girls, who slammed desks and broke wind into the reverberant canvas-and-metal chairs during assembly. He left to become headmaster of a famous school in North Yorkshire.

My new school produced few notable alumni. There was a quiet young man who became Britain's first black police chief constable, a fellow who sparkled briefly as a boxer before fizzling, and a sad weed of a boy who finished up behind bars as one of the country's most notorious child murderers.

I was terrified of being late for school so I would arrive very early and as soon as the doors were unlocked I would help arrange the chairs in the hall. The task was repetitious and systematic.

Nobody spoke. This regimentation calmed me down. Things were under control.

They had put me in the top stream but it wasn't long before the trouble started. My maths teacher Mr Bird found it impossible to accept my profound inability to grasp the basics. After a week of long division we had a test. I just couldn't do it.

'But we did this *yesterday*,' shouted Mr Bird. I was too dismayed to reply.

At home, I tried to explain to my father: 'As soon as I'm onto the second bit I've forgotten the first bit. And the numbers look as if they are jumping about.' My dad looked at me strangely.

Temple Grandin says that despite her brilliance in other subjects her brain's 'math department' is 'trashed'. I couldn't have put it better myself. There is actually a fancy name for this: 'dyscalculia'. I shan't be using it again.

The problem, which nobody understood, including me, was that the maths bucket of my brain was actually a sieve: strong on the slow sifting and qualitative analysis of information — finding likenesses and differences, identifying weaknesses, spotting fundamentals — but extravagantly weak at rapid filling and storage. My short-term memory was lousy. Maths just wasn't my thing, and shouting '*We did this yesterday*' was not the answer.

Mr Bird demanded my demotion to a lower stream but several of my teachers objected. IQ tests were done on me and I scored lower than expected. Mr Bird felt vindicated.

'The boy is not very bright,' he said.

'Have you *spoken* to him?' responded my biology teacher in disbelief.

Hans Asperger himself coined the term 'autistic intelligence', which he said had distinct qualities and was the opposite of conventional learning and worldly-wise cunning. It is difficult to measure the IQ of an autistic person, who may well not want to communicate, or cooperate, or either, skipping questions that do not appeal, or spoiling the ballot paper by answering arbitrarily.

This general disinclination to comply is profound in autism, and extends from the meal table and school classroom to adult employment, where otherwise technically adept Aspergers are likely to find jobs and bosses so difficult that they become deeply miserable and sometimes unemployable. This fact is shockingly unappreciated by many schoolteachers, examiners, university interviewers, and employers, who insist on dismissing fish who fail to run, while neglecting to test their swimming ability.

I clung on in the top stream but the maths never improved.

One thing I could do was draw. I would sit for hours engrossed by a human skull or piece of driftwood, whose fissures and ridges I would painstakingly transcribe in line. A large fearless boy called Mick was impressed by my drawings, and my ability to make him laugh with my strange sense of humour. 'If anyone tries to beat you up,' he said, 'tell me and I'll smash their face in.' It was a reassuring relationship.

Mick's mother ran a newsagent's and once embarrassed herself by calling a customer whose name was Mrs Polly 'Mrs Parrott'. His father had been a nightclub drummer and boasted of tapping out rhythms for the New York stripper Gypsy Rose Lee. He was the only man I have ever seen who shook curry powder on his food, like pepper. Mick left school early with the ambition of joining the army and, he told me, travelling the globe on a huge motorbike with a naked Miss World riding pillion.

I was never bullied at school, except by the occasional teacher. To deflect aggression I used avoidance first, and then, if necessary, humour. All the same, boys would yell out rude comments, because I often looked odd, in an old-fashioned way. I had long Pre-Raphaelite hair and, outside of school, habitually wore corduroy jackets and unfashionable footwear such as suede shoes, or sandals with socks, which unnerved my anxious sister Rebecca. Not so long ago I read that the writer and broadcaster Garrison Keillor had identified himself as being on the autism spectrum. I immediately remembered the peculiar sandals he insists on wearing.

★

One day my dad told me that there had been an outbreak of water pistols at the school where he taught. The teachers had confiscated them and as they were comparing differing models in the staffroom one of them idly squirted a colleague, accidentally on purpose. 'That's your game, is it!' said the man, leaping behind a chair and flourishing his own weapon. Within seconds it was like *The Battle of the Century*, with teachers, male and female, screaming with laughter as they drenched each other with their confiscated firearms.

I was chuckling about this as I walked home for lunch. Unusually, my mother was in the house. She looked grave.

'Your father's been in a crash,' she said. 'He was hit by a car and he's in hospital. They think his lung has collapsed. It's touch and go.'

I didn't know what I was supposed to do.

'Oh,' I said. 'Better eat my lunch.'

I loved my dad, but the emotion just didn't come out, and my mother, full of understandable anxiety, was hurt and confused by my apparent lack of empathy for my dad, and for her.

From an evolutionary viewpoint it must be important for at

least some group members not to go to pieces in a disaster, though more demonstrative people probably find this hard to admire.

I am reminded of an Aspergic teenager, the friend of a friend, who was nearly killed when a car hit his bike from the side. When my friend went to see him in hospital she found him plugged into various bits of kit, his face purple and black. He looked up at her with bloodshot eyes but didn't smile or hold out his arms to greet her. Through swollen lips he said, 'Do you have any questions you wish to ask about my injuries?'

My dad had broken several bones, one of which had punctured his lung, and his motorbike was a tangled write-off. But he came home after a bit and made a complete, very lucky, recovery.

★

They made us learn ballroom dancing at school. The man who taught us was a grey cadaver named Mr Buerk, known to us as 'The Berk'. To the accompaniment of *The Blue Danube* and the *Radetzky March* squawking out of an old record player, he would swirl Miss Swanepoel, the typing teacher, around the disinfectancy-smelling school gym while we uncoordinated teenagers shambled about in extreme embarrassment, holding our partners like bags of radioactive waste.

The Berk drove a Land Rover covered in wartime camouflage netting, and once took out a Luger pistol which he waved around, claiming to have taken it from the body of a Nazi soldier who he said he had strangled, commando style. On another occasion he handed out some foolscap posters bearing the logotype of the National Front and emblazoned with a slogan about 'jungle bunnies'. 'If anyone asks where you got them,' said The Berk, sliding a dry palm across his Brilliantined hair, 'say you found them in a telephone box. That's the trick.'

Shortly after this, the corner shop run by Mr Singh received through its window a half-brick marked 'NF'. When the police came knocking at The Berk's nearby house, five pubescent boys were spotted escaping shirtless over the back fence and he found himself fairly smartly a guest of Her Majesty.

But the people I loathed most at school were the games masters. There was a rotund unmarried homunculus called Robbins who smelt of carbolic soap and had a forest of hair growing out of his ears. He would come into the changing rooms and viciously flick naked boys with a wet towel. Then there was Mr Nundy, a muscle-bound dunce who used to throw into the mud any boy not thoroughly filthy after a game of rugby.

I hated sport but found myself volunteered into an after-school judo club, a frightening world of rubber smells, squeaks, shouting echoes, special clothes that made my skin crawl, and other people touching me. I lasted one session.

The school was on the site of an old farm and on its outskirts was a decaying barn to which we were often ordered to run during PE lessons. One day on the way to the barn I found myself being overtaken by the fattest and slowest boys. Soon they had rounded the building and were on their way back. I was achingly fatigued, panting hard, and spitting a fiery yellow substance. I realised I wasn't going to make it and turned back, the rest of the boys passing me on their return journey, yelling jovial insults as I stumbled exhausted back to the changing rooms.

I had been feeling rotten for some time. I was losing weight, had a constant dry-mouthed thirst, and was getting up to pee several times a night. My mother took me to see Dr Armstrong.

'I'm going to issue a carbohydrate challenge,' he said. 'Go away, eat a whole packet of Jaffa Cakes, and come back in an hour.'

Back in the surgery he performed some alchemy on my urine, dropping a fat tablet into a test tube, where it fizzed for a minute before ominously changing colour.

'It's diagnostic,' he said to my mother. 'Diabetes.'

'We'll get you into hospital this afternoon,' he told me, 'You'll be on insulin for the rest of your life.'

I have now had type-1 diabetes for nearly half a century and have given myself something like 45,000 injections, but though this has been a huge part of every one of my days it is a story for a different book. All I will say is that having Asperger's syndrome as well as diabetes has been the greatest blessing. No two conditions could be better matched. My non-stop nit-picking and rigid focus on detail and rules have made me monitor my blood glucose and insulin levels so vigilantly that I have managed to avoid the serious complications that visit havoc upon the lives of many longstanding diabetics.

The other thing is that my Aspergic resistance to complying with advice from unimaginative and occasionally silly nurses and doctors has allowed me to invent my own eccentric but effective ways of dealing with the condition. My endocrinologist once asked me how I kept my diabetes under such good control.

'I don't pay any attention to my doctors,' I told him.

'That's it!' he said. 'We want people to take control themselves.'

Control has always been a big thing for me.

★

In the summer holidays of 1975, I spent a season with the National Youth Theatre in London. The NYT was the brainchild of the writer and sometime schoolteacher Michael Croft, a big man with an appetite for plays, grub, life, and booze. Someone called him a Falstaff with a family of Prince Hals and he certainly had a way with young men, who often found themselves invited back to his pad in North London for a glass of something.

Each year Croft put on three or four plays at the Shaw Theatre in St Pancras, with a company of aspirant actors. Something like three thousand youngsters auditioned each season, but unlike most of the hopefuls I didn't want to act, I wanted to do set design, which might be how I got in.

The actors were based at the theatre while those of us doing the sets had to travel to a vast workshop and scenery store in St Katherine Docks near the Tower of London. I commuted daily from home and late at night there were often elderly tarts and other dodgy characters loitering around the dockers' pubs or at Victoria station.

At fifteen, I was, I think, the youngest of the class of 1975. I was also the only one of the handful of us doing set design who was not secretly an actor who had failed his audition.

I was frequently sent to deliver things, or to measure stuff backstage in the silent theatre. I remember once coming out into the alley beyond the stage door, where a smelly old female tramp shouted 'Arse'oles!' at me. Being a prim little thing I was quite shocked. Another time I remember being overawed by the presence of the old music hall comedian and actor Max Wall, who had a show on at the theatre. He was sitting in the bar alone, with a face like a seaside town in the rain.

In the prop cupboard I recall a rack of stage champagne with a faint grey notice across its label: 'This bottle contains LEMONADE', and sealed containers of stage blood, known as 'Kensington Gore'. It was a great delight to spend time in the quiet behind the scenes.

I was good at lettering and one afternoon Michael Croft spotted me backstage preparing a poster for *Henry IV, part I*. He asked me upstairs into his office above the auditorium.

'Shut the door,' he said.

I looked at him across the big room. He had an unfathomable expression on his face and I was immediately alert.

'What's your name?' he asked, looking me up and down.

'Thomas Cutler,' I said, giving it to him in full in an effort to make myself appear larger.

'How old are you?'

'Fifteen.'

Croft smiled an inscrutable smile.

'Go on. Off you go,' he said kindly.

Naive, autistic, and passive as I was, I didn't know quite what was going on, though I knew it was something.

Though I enjoyed my time backstage I have never been much good as a member of a theatre audience. It's dark and there are people close to me, sniffing and twisting. I remember going to the Roundhouse in 1976 to see Peter Brook's production of *The Ik*, where the throat clearing was worse than an outing of the National Pleurisy Society. It's the same in cinemas and concert halls, where a cough, often as loud as a mezzo forte blast on the French horn, causes in me a battened-down fury out of all proportion. I prefer to watch films and listen to music at home, on my own.

My music teacher Mr George was a white-haired Scot with stubby fingers and a tweed suit. He had pushed a piano over the Cairngorms and claimed it was this, rather than his twenty-a-day Capstan-Full-Strength habit, that had given him heart disease. You could make up a tune, hum it to Mr George at the keyboard, and he would immediately harmonise it in whatever style you chose, from

Bay City Rollers to Beethoven. He knew I played the guitar and encouraged me to study an orchestral instrument. I chose the double bass, which never really suited me. I got as far as *The Elephant* by Saint-Saëns, but found the close proximity of a lot of other people in an orchestra a recipe for high anxiety.

Discos and rock festivals were always a terrifying idea, and indeed I have never been to one of either. I feared the darkness and the noise, the thumping music. The press of all those people disturbed me, like a Nuremberg rally. So it was strange that I should accept a ticket for *Top of the Pops*.

A BBC producer had asked a few of us from my school to contribute to a mild TV documentary and the *Top of the Pops* tickets were a thank-you. I have always been completely unaware of popular culture. I had no idea who was in the Rolling Stones or what was number one in the hit parade, and my growing record collection contained a lot of weird stuff, including fairground organs, musical boxes, and several sound effects records. Sound effects is still one of my enthusiasms. Visiting *Top of the Pops* I felt like an anthropologist examining an undiscovered tribe.

The show was recorded in a surprisingly small studio at BBC Television Centre, where the sets were noticeably grubby, torn, and dented, though on screen everything looked glamorous and twinkly. The performers on the night included Bryan Ferry, Nat King Cole's daughter Natalie Cole, and a man calling himself Gilbert O'Sullivan, all miming to loud playback coming out of a plywood speaker that was rolled around on battered wheels.

Before the recording, the crowd was given a strict talking to by a man with a horrible face. 'If a camera is moving towards you get out of the way because he won't stop.' In the event, this advice was academic, since striding in front of the camera came a bear of a man who simply pushed people aside. But the most important admonition seemed to be this: 'WE DON'T WANT MEN DANCING TOGETHER. NO MEN DANCING TOGETHER. UNDERSTOOD? NO! MEN! DANCING! TOGETHER!' After a while it sank in.

Since ballroom dancing with The Berk I have never danced, and find the idea disturbing. This has sometimes wounded my wife, as well as a couple of other young ladies who approached me at various weddings and things and resented being rebuffed. Thank God at *Top of the Pops* I wasn't forced to. I positioned myself instead on the edge of the swarm, out of shot: the watcher in the shadows, assessing the expertise of the camera operators and other technicians and analysing the way the programme was being put together.

When I later watched the show at home with my family I spotted the back of my head being briefly mixed into a shot of the female dancing group known as Pan's People, who on television looked very sexy but who in real life were sweating and grunting like horses, behind Pan Am smiles. It was another lesson that the way things looked was not necessarily the way things were.

★

Gordon Parkhurst was a curly haired youth who, like me, was good at art. Gordon had an enviable way with girls and one day showed me the first pornographic magazine I had ever seen. It contained a gaudy picture of a lady with her pubic hair shaved off, to which he drew my particular attention. On another occasion he followed our young teacher Miss Legge into the art room stock cupboard, closing the door behind him. There was the sound of softly clinking jam jars before Miss Legge emerged, cheeks flushed, smoothing down her skirt.

My friend Jon and I were starting our A-level studies and we asked if we could have a life-drawing class at school. Miss Legge put it to the higher-ups who ummed and ahed before nervously agreeing, with the proviso that this was an experiment open only to pupils already doing art. And so money was found — I think our parents chipped in — the windows of the art room were papered over, and the young model arrived, undressing as required behind a screen. Even though we were seventeen, with all the hormones going at full blast, the mood in the room always resembled that of a class of respectful anatomists examining a cadaver. Models became personally attractive only once they were dressed again. As far as I know, this was the first time that pupils in an English school had been permitted to draw live naked women.

If you were aiming for art college you were expected to do A-level art history. Our art history teacher, silver-haired Mr Lutyens, had been at the Royal College with Lucian Freud, John Minton, and other well-knowns, and regaled us with rude tales about his time there. We particularly enjoyed his impression of a very camp Francis Bacon having a sulk.

A-level English was less amusing. They made us read *Jude the Obscure*, which I found unbearably gloomy, and I was the only one in the class who seemed not to have grasped, or be interested in, the idea that the fog so elaborately described at the beginning of *Bleak House* was a metaphor for the law. Literary metaphors of this kind often go over my head.

Like other Aspergers, I have never been much of a novel reader. I don't seem to get the same thrill from novels as your average book lover. This tendency in readers with Asperger's has often been noted and a possible reason for it was revealed in a 2016 report in the Royal Society journal *Open Science Experiments*, which found that fiction causes the body to release pain-killing endorphins and promotes social bonding, an effect seen also in laughing, singing, and dancing. Whether unsmiling, non-dancing, non-singing Aspergers fail to get the same chemical rewards from fiction as other more socially bonded people is the subject for somebody's PhD.

My favourite books were biographies, exhibition catalogues, and texts on typography and magic. Amongst the fiction I did like were ghost stories and detective mysteries, including the *Maigret* novellas by Georges Simenon, and Raymond Chandler's Philip Marlowe adventures. These were generally shorter and more concrete than the novels I found such sterile going.

One day my father gave me a copy of *The Hound of the Baskervilles* by Arthur Conan Doyle. I read *this* novel with enormous relish and it affected me so much that Sherlock Holmes and his world became my new enthusiasm. I got hold of all the Sherlock Holmes adventures, four novels and fifty-six short stories, and soon knew them inside out.

★

I was a late developer and did not yet realise that at heart I was a writer myself. From an early age I had had a bent for the geometry and mechanics of language. I saw linguistic communication as an engineering job and had a knack for identifying the crucial architecture of a sentence, just as an engineer might pick out the vital members of an iron bridge. I had always enjoyed parsing sentences, which we did in English when I was twelve, until modern teaching precepts swept the idea away.

I took a delight in wordplay, and the straitjacket of limericks and palindromes particularly appealed. 'Satan oscillate my metallic sonatas!' seemed to me as good as anything by T. S. Eliot, whose name I noticed was an anagram of 'toilets'.

When a German exchange student came to stay he said I was the only person whose English he could readily understand. I seemed to have a natural grasp of the best method of getting my meaning across. First you had to abandon idiom. 'I'm popping up the road', 'Do you need to spend a penny?', or 'He has ideas above his station' were the kinds of things that people would come out with, causing deep furrows to form in the brows of their foreign interlocutors. In speaking English to the French, or Spanish, or Italian you had to make sure to use plenty of long words, which tend to have their roots in Latin and are therefore more easily guessable by speakers of these Romance languages than short words rooted in the Anglo-Frisian dialects of Old English. In describing a potter's vase, 'ceramic' is a better word than 'clay'.

It was a bit different with the Germans, where syntax was the vital thing. In putting together a sentence 'the words or members, most nearly related, should be placed as near to each other as possible,' as the grammarian Lindley Murray put it in 1795.

My German teacher was Mr Evans, a mummified creature who had never been abroad and had a distaste for modern languages. He would take out his pill bottles in class and encourage us to sniff the uncanny odour of the cotton wool. He drove an improbable sports car full of torn exercise books and trailing wires. To start it he had to take a battery from the boot, stagger to the front, lift the bonnet and attach jump leads, before humping it back to the boot again. He went through this magnetic performance every day for years. The idea of having the car repaired seemed not to have occurred to him. Mr Evans taught me almost no German but an enormous amount about what life could do to you.

My French teacher Mr Zamenhof was a Pole with dyed-purple hair and a fuzzy number on his forearm. Known as 'Chopper Zamenhof', he ran French Club at lunchtime, where he made a delicious version of coffee, using evaporated milk. Anybody who misbehaved would be threatened with his notorious karate move, known as 'The Chop', and treated to a string of heavily accented abuse: 'Dirty, ugly, naughty little one — *fly* from French Club!' Mr Zamenhof once accidentally locked Mme Bonnard in the stock cupboard. One day I saw him parked in town behind the wheel of his car. He was weeping in great gasps. His whole family had gone up in smoke in the camps.

It seemed necessary to have a girlfriend, and on my way to school I spotted a dark-eyed creature called Katy. It wasn't just a girl's prettiness that made her attractive — it was her confidence, and her intelligence. Katy was full of aplomb. She was a very good pianist, spoke French, and had a delicious laugh. Her sunny outlook counterbalanced my reserve. Her parents lived in a small house with no books in it and her eye was on the horizon. She told me she planned to visit Rome to learn Italian before going to London University to study English. I had no idea what my plans were, beyond trying to get into some art school or other.

I was no good at flirting, flowers, and romance. Nonetheless restaurants and pubs were visited, cinemas patronised, and walks taken. I found it hard to read the signals but in due course, and after a good deal of hard work on my part, the vertical progressed to the horizontal.

First love is often steeped in meaning but I made far too much of it all, turning Katy into my new 'special interest' hang-up. My expectations were astronomically high and the intensity of my attachment, known to nobody but myself, was out of all proportion.

Perfect commitment is too much to expect of anybody, let alone a determined young woman with a string of books under her arm and the itch to get away.

Katy visited Italy as she had said she would and rang me from there. Afterwards she gave me a copy of *Strait Is the Gate* by André Gide, the story of a sensitive boy deeply in love with a girl — with whom, he is sure, his life will be forever entwined — as she goes deliberately and inexorably cold. My literal self refused to get the message, and it is only writing about it today, forty years later, that I have finally taken the hint. Though now it is more than too late.

I tried to hold things together but Katy's vaulting ambition was more ardent even than my own lust for perfection. 'You treat me like a thing,' she said. It ended. I don't think I ever got over it. Only recently have I learnt, to my great great relief, that such quixotic overbearing attachments are a classic hallmark of the Asperger self.

In 2017, naturalist Chris Packham presented a BBC Television programme about his life with Asperger's, during which he described his boyhood infatuation with a kestrel. 'I loved it with an enormous passion and amount of energy … The obsessive interest and intense focus on that one organism meant that I could just exclude everything else. All that existed was just us two … I don't think that I've ever loved anything as intensely.' But after a few 'perfect' months the bird died, an event Packham described as, 'catastrophic' and, 'an enormous turning point'. All this struck a resounding chord with me. Such monomania does not bring contentment.

One morning I looked into the mirror. My left shoulder and the side of my neck were peppered with angry spots. Dr Armstrong took one look: 'Under stress?'

'A levels coming up,' I said. I didn't mention Katy.

'It's shingles,' he said. 'Go straight home and go to bed. If it reaches that eye, we could be in trouble.'

Days and nights passed in a haze. I was feverish. A breeze blowing across the now hideous rash was unbearable. Interviews with various art schools were in the diary. Jon offered to assemble my portfolio.

After a time, things began to improve, but there was still a feathery electric pain in my skin. Even today if a shirt brushes across the pale splotches left by the rash it makes me gasp.

I dragged myself and my portfolio off to several London art colleges. At the Slade, Sir Lawrence Gowing, an ungainly stuttering giant, dribbled over my life drawings.

'You ah ah ah did these ats ats — at school?'

'Yes,' I said.

'These are ah ah ah — they're very good.'

I looked blank. Nobody had told me about selling yourself. It was the age *before* selling yourself and I was terribly naive. Every other applicant had done a foundation year and already looked like an artist. I was dressed in a jacket and tie, straight out of the Asperger's wardrobe. I felt lost. They told me to do a foundation course and they'd have me next year. I was too young.

The Central School of Art were so impressed they offered me a place *without* the expected foundation year. 'That's unheard of,' said Miss Legge, but I turned them down, pinning my hopes instead on my first-choice university, which was one of a handful doing a practical Fine Art degree course. Learning that I had said no the Central School Miss Legge blew her top, telling me that I'd made a gigantic mistake. I scoffed. How could I know that she was right and I was wrong? Just how wrong I would come to find out.

But something else was amiss. I felt as though a surgeon had opened my head. People appeared to be speaking in slow motion.

My hands were unusual, and I had become increasingly uncommunicative. Everybody's talk was of exams, but I could hardly move. My obvious collapse inward seemed inexplicable to my teachers. My parents received the final report from my form master: 'Tom sits alone, silent, lost in a world of his own.'

When the exams came round there were problems. I became tremendously distracted during the art history paper. The room stank of food and the timekeeper kept writing a cricket score on a blackboard at the front, leaving me endlessly dreading the next interruption and the mind-blowing screech of chalk. Someone somewhere was sniffing. Over and over the desk of the girl two rows ahead of me kept squealing, like a monkey caught in a trap.

The English paper had a question that read: 'In *Bleak House* character spins the plot. Comment.' I was flummoxed. 'Spins the plot'? What did *that* mean? What *did* that mean? And who cared about characters? Not me. If they had asked me to write about Dickens' handling of paragraph transitions in building a narrative, or chapter architecture in serial publication, I could have done something. But I didn't understand what they wanted, and wasn't interested. Instead I wrote a withering critique of the question, pointing out its faults.

In all the years I'd been at school nobody had ever explained that exams ought not to be taken to heart. They were a game that, once you understood the rules, could be laughed off rather easily. In my rigid, moralistic naivety I believed that the real point here was higher-quality question setting, so I said so. I wasn't going to play games. The trouble was that, as the Chinese sage pointed out, it was a false economy to burn down your house in order to inconvenience your mother-in-law.

I waited for my results. On some days I couldn't get up. On better days I would sit alone, slowly practising second deals beside the blue cones of the blossoming buddleia. I was a ghost. I was lost, and by the wind grieved.

When it came in, the news was bad. I'd got a D in art, my main subject, and I didn't just fail English I got a U, standing for 'Unclassified', meaning 'unclassifiably bad'. I did okay in art history.

My parents demanded a review. The examination board came back, defending the marking. In art, we were told, 'form cannot be described in line alone'. As my drawings were exclusively line drawings this unbargained-for commandment rendered several years' work futile, as it must have done for Picasso, Matisse, Hockney, Warhol, and the vase painters of Ancient Greece.

At the time I didn't understand, but now I know, that you will never be any good at passing exams if you fail to conform, since part of their job is to discipline the wayward and the recusant.

Miss Legge said she would take things further, but coming down the A285 one evening a lorry went into her, and that was that. It was academic anyway because, based, rather amusingly, on their great admiration for my line drawings, my first-choice university had only asked for two Es. I had scraped in.

The groves of academe beckoned. I was to be off, out into the world, leaving home for the first time. I thought back over my schooldays. I remembered Iain Westmore who'd drunk two pints of eggnog in a domestic science lesson and vomited prodigiously into the girls' toilets; I recalled the pretty student teacher who had sat on a collapsible trestle table in the art room and fallen over backwards, exposing her knickers; I remembered Mr George pushing a piano over the Cairngorms, cigarette in mouth, and Mr Robbins with his wet towel, flicking naked buttocks in the showers. I tried to forget, but could not forget, Katy.

I understood nothing about myself, and nothing about the

world. I was empty: my body a seedless shell, yet inside something was chasing me. Where was I going? Formless weather systems swirled around and I could not escape the Big Question, the one to which the Church said it had the answer: *What was the point?* Maybe Van Gogh had had the right idea. Maybe oblivion was the way out.

Though I didn't know it I was in the grip of a very serious depression. Had there been a magic wand on the table with the power to wave away my misery, I could not have been bothered to pick it up. *For the thing which I greatly feared was come upon me, and that which I was afraid of was come unto me. I was not in safety, neither had I rest, neither was I quiet; yet trouble came.*

Chapter 4:
Steep hill upwards

The one thing we can never get enough of is love.
And the one thing we never give enough of is love.

HENRY MILLER

Autumn was unusually sunny and warm that year. As the days shortened, the practical preparations for moving out occupied my thoughts.

When the day came that my father was to drive me to the university, we made an early start. In the passenger seat sat my mother, rotating the map on her knee and telling Dad when he had gone the wrong way or chosen the wrong gear. 'You're in third, you know,' she would say as he negotiated a tricky roundabout or tried to accelerate onto a motorway. I was squashed in the back with my student baggage — artist's materials, books, LPs, rusting bicycle — watching from the rear window as my past unrolled from the vehicle's cloaca in an improbable ribbon.

The ancient minster town we were heading for stood at the confluence of two rivers. The ruins of a flint abbey occupied a central plot, its last dissident abbot having been hung, drawn, and quartered in front of his church. Once important, the town had lost much of its grandeur, its modern history being one of brewing and biscuit manufacture. The university was not prestigious, its most famous products being a number of television weather-forecasters and the robotic seat used on his television show by the creepy child molester Jimmy Savile.

Owing to some bungle, no place had been found for me in any of the student halls of residence dotted about the university. Instead I was to be put up in the suburbs by a middle-aged couple, Mr and Mrs Chambers. We arrived at the house, pleasantries were exchanged, my stuff was unloaded, and I waved my parents off.

Dressed in a protective blue tabard Mrs Chambers showed me round. She drew my attention to some framed photographs of her children wearing academic gowns and clasping certificates. She indicated the hi-fi equipment, on the lid of which was a record sleeve. 'Moon Over Naples', it said. She showed me the three-piece suite, an antimacassar over the back of each armchair, and asked me to use a drinks coaster. She showed me the cornflakes in the kitchen cupboard and pointed out what she called the 'conveniences'. From the lip of the toilet bowl hung a small plastic cage containing a chemical block that turned the water blue when you operated the flush. To camouflage the horror of the spare toilet roll on the cistern Mrs Chambers had placed a crocheted dairymaid over it. Everything in the house was spotless. There wasn't a book to be seen.

'Mr Chambers will be home at five fifteen and he will take you to the pub,' said Mrs Chambers, spraying furniture polish at a glazed print of a mountain sunset. Her premonition proved accurate and on the dot I spotted through the modesty glass of the front door the distorted form of Mr Chambers shimmering down the path.

After exchanging his blue trilby for a beige one he walked us to his local, where he bought me half a pint of sterilised beer and sat us down on a severely upholstered bench. Between the horse brasses, various Rotary Club notices announced forthcoming charitable dos. Mr Chambers spoke softly so as not to disturb the other merrymakers, who sat in nylon blazers beside the hissing plastic-coal fire looking as though life had dealt them hands of disappointment and defeat.

'They make you feel very hospitable here,' fumbled Mr Chambers, removing a particle of dust from the gleaming table with the corner of a starched handkerchief. It was as if his mind had been flushed clean by a blue chemical block.

There was no teaching at the university yet. Instead, something called freshers' week was under way and everyone was registering, picking up timetables, choosing subsidiary courses, and finding their way about the campus. We had been encouraged to visit the freshers' fair, an induction event taking place at the students' union, the place, it was said, where you went to strike up new friendships, buy a scarf in the university colours, or ask for help if you were going bonkers.

The freshers' fair turned out to be a ramshackle event, with representatives of assorted clubs, from beekeeping, to history, to gay, sitting behind trestle tables around the walls of what was apparently some sort of dance hall or dining hall. Depending on just where you stood, the place smelt of shepherd's pie or pineapple urinal deodorisers. Here and there hooray henrys in striped shirts handed out rugby leaflets, new students chatted to other new students, and predatory agents of the various churches smiled at you competitively. Under a wisp of bunting someone was trying to recruit aspiring journalists to the student newspaper. A headline on its front page showed that the bar had been set low: 'Cybernetics annex flat roof "prone to leaks" says student'.

I had never been to a freshers' fair and, though everybody else appeared to know what was going on and what to do, I was at a loss. The rooms were lit by fluorescent lights, there were many people, and the hullabaloo was intense.

The walls seemed to be inching in on me so I made my way to the upstairs bar, which at this time of day was dark and quiet. The carpet smelt wonderfully of sour beer. I ordered a pint and sat down on my own in a musty corner. On the table was a cheaply printed leaflet. 'Would you like to help us start a university radio station?' it said. Radio was something I was keen on. I had always fiddled about with reel-to-reel tape recorders and microphones and I loved to listen to radio features on the BBC. I had been captivated by *Plain Tales from the Raj*, a series of programmes featuring stories of British India told by the people who were there. I admired the birdlike skill with which the producer had systematically assembled each episode from thousands of little pieces.

I was also deeply impressed by the poetic-montage features of a radio producer called, rather wonderfully, Piers Plowright. His haunting programme on the subject of death I have never forgotten.

Since the age of thirteen I had made a recording every year of the Christmas *Festival of Nine Lessons and Carols* from King's College, Cambridge, which was broadcast live on the radio. After editing out the Bible readings, which I knew almost by heart, I would transfer the carols to a cassette tape. I continued recording the broadcasts until the demise of cassettes, when, with a heavy heart, I threw out more than thirty years' worth.

A related interest was sound effects, in which I took a great pleasure. I would annoy my family during episodes of *Columbo* by saying things like 'Footsteps wrong as usual' or 'Funny how the sound of the closing front door is exactly the same as the bedroom door'. At other times I would announce, 'That cat meowing is from *BBC Sound Effects*, LP 4, band 7a.' I once gave a talk on the subject at school, to the frank bemusement and, I imagine, deep boredom of the class, for whom such details were irrelevant.

Just a Minute was a BBC radio comedy panel game that I greatly enjoyed. At that time it was taped in a former underground cinema in Lower Regent Street identifiable on the radio by the occasional rumble of Tube trains. I went to many of these recordings while I was at school and once saw the music hall comedian Tommy Trinder make a guest appearance. Among the regular contributors were the actor–impresario Derek Nimmo, who always arrived in his chauffeur-driven Rolls Royce; the chef-cum-MP Clement Freud, who tended to dismiss fans with a backhand brush-off; and Kenneth Williams, the actor, raconteur, and diarist. Unlike Freud, Williams was charm itself, especially with children, for whom he clearly had remarkable respect.

I slipped the leaflet about the new university radio station into my pocket.

Freshers' week continued to pass slowly in a muddle of library tours, solitary pizza meals, a talk from the gowned sub-dean about the love of learning for its own sake, and a growing feeling that I had fallen down Alice's rabbit hole. I spoke to almost nobody.

As an insulin-controlled diabetic it was important for me to sign up with a doctor to arrange my prescriptions so I went along to the university medical centre, which had a tank of warm-water fish in its reception and its own cottage-hospital-type ward upstairs. There were leaflets about VD, and posters asking for healthy student volunteers for a 'research project'. A bearded fellow with his leg in a cast told me, 'I did that. It's money for nothing. All you do is masturbate into a yoghurt pot.' It sounded a ridiculous way to make a living.

We had been told to report our presence to the art department. Art being perceived, possibly, as an 'unclean' subject, the department was situated on a separate site half an hour from the main campus. It was a pleasant stroll down the steep hill, past the Edwardian terraces and the hospital where Douglas Bader had had his legs amputated.

Like the main campus, this one was entirely self-contained. Enclosed by monastic shrub-sheathed cloisters was the sharply trimmed lawn of a central quadrangle. Off the quad were two or three departments, including art and food science, a subject that I never quite understood though I think it has something to do with the development of chemically engineered cheese and extruded snacks.

I walked the cloisters, a circuit I was to take many times over the next few years, till I reached the department's administrative section: two or three offices clustered behind a pair of rickety double doors smeared with the painty finger marks of bygone students. In one of these rooms sat a secretary. I stepped forward, submitted my details, and a box was ticked.

The Professor of Fine Art was to give an introductory talk and an excited gaggle were arranging themselves about the studio on clattering metal chairs. Distant echoes of last term's linseed oil filled the air and everybody but me was dressed in paint-splashed over-alls. Most, for some reason, were wearing builders' boots. They all smoked roll-ups, a club badge like the crest on Mr Chambers' blazer pocket. In my jacket and V-neck sweater I must have looked like a representative of the local golf club.

The professor was a ghostly presence, so lukewarm that I remember almost nothing he ever said, though I do recollect the smell of his pipe smoke, which filled the corridors whenever he was there. He did no teaching that I recall.

After his trifling introduction we were spoken to by one of the lecturers who came up on the train from London most days to supervise the teaching of first-year students. This man was Austin Randall, a painter just out of his twenties who had been a student in the same department not long before. A tall figure with a hunch, Austin smoked incessant roll-ups, had brown dirt under his fingernails, and spoke with a distinctive whistly delivery. He often seemed to be going somewhere with what he was saying but the trouble was that when he got there you wondered why he had bothered. 'There'sss sssixsss sssortsss of ssshapesss, I sssupossse,' he said, 'and sssixsss sssortsss of sssurfacccesss.' Many students took such fatuities for pearls of wisdom. Austin's paintings looked to me like occupational therapy.

Playing Robin to Austin's Batman was a young woman called Fleeta Swit, who detested me from the start. As I would learn, Fleeta, like Austin, expected students to paint in a style resembling as closely as possible her own. She produced an unvarying stream of brightly coloured circles and squares, and if you decided that you might have an idea of your own — having been drawing and painting since you were a boy — you were shot down in flames. At the time I impugned, and I still impugn, the seriousness of Austin

179

and Fleeta as teachers, as painters, and as people.

The best painter in the university was a man called Terry Frost, who had the titles Artist in Residence and Professor of Painting. He had a grey military moustache and zingy clothes, and was great friends with Roger Hilton and Mark Rothko. Frost was the only artist I have ever met who seriously wore a beret. He also wore huge spectacles that made him look like my grandmother. His work was beautiful and he made no qualitative distinction between figurative and abstract art, excelling in both. His paintings revealed those of Fleeta Swit to be frail derivations.

Terry Frost had a favourite aphorism. 'Life's a bowl of cherries,' he would say, and he said it often. Sometimes I felt he was saying it because he couldn't think of anything else to say. He was a great family man and years later his son Stephen Frost would make his name as a comedian.

The most intellectually interesting member of staff was Tony the technician, a practical man with grown-up children. His job was to help around the rabbit warren of studios, which were divided up by year. He put up partitions between one student painter and the next, or fixed things that broke. I spoke to Tony as he prepared my space by erecting panels and securing them to the floor. 'I've been here fourteen years,' he told me, a nail between his teeth, 'and I've seen everything. The first year exhibition: really interesting, it all looks exciting and different. Second year: less so. Third year: hard to tell one painter from the next. Final show: everything exactly the same.' Tony was Professor Emeritus of Having Your Head Screwed On and I think he alone amongst the staff noticed that there was something awry in me.

Among the new students were two Bobs. Bob Strange was aptly named. He dressed very oddly and had a pudding bowl haircut and vast unflattering glasses. His portfolio was full of drawings of classical sculpture. He smoked miniature cigars, which he would pierce with a cocktail stick when they shrank too small to hold with the fingers, enabling him to suck out the final minim of goodness.

Possibly because he was strange, Bob was one of the few people who did speak to me. One day he showed me a stick of chalky pastel. 'It's called sanguine,' he said earnestly, looking slightly crackers, 'It produces a blood-red line.' He had unusual fixations, on one occasion showing me a pamphlet about a dead Catholic friar who was said to have had bleeding lesions on his hands corresponding with the crucifixion wounds of Jesus Christ. I was sceptical; he didn't push it.

The other Bob was Bob Scotland: tall and tremendously self-confident, with no boundary between his chest hair and the stubble that darkened his chin twenty minutes after he had shaved. In one incomprehensible exercise that we were made to do, a huge roll of paper was pinned along a wall and we were instructed each to paint a vertical line on it. I made the tiniest mark I could, up near a corner. Bob Scotland splashed a four-foot-wide black strip down the middle, obliterating the lines of many of the other students.

The weeks passed. Everybody else seemed at ease. They compared paintbrushes, chatted, or invited each other to parties. Before long some were arriving in the studios hand in hand.

I was feeling strange. Though used to my own company, I hadn't made proper human contact for too long and the hard edges of the days made me long for some softness. I eyed various girls in the studio. They seemed either unavailable or unattractive. There was Bernice: rather masculine and gruff in her denim fisherman's smock, always smoking; there was Big Lil, who drank pints and had a huge face; there was pretty Sue, who, when I tried to say something amusing, rounded on me, catching me completely off guard. 'What the *hell*,' she snapped, 'is that supposed to mean?!' What had I said wrong? My favourite was a beautiful young woman called Alice, with strawberry blonde hair and a terrific smile. But she was going out with, and presumably staying in with, a fellow from the typography department, the son of a man who read out the news on television. Each time I tried to catch her eye she blanked me. The position was hopeless. I wondered what Katy was doing. I was homesick.

That evening, I returned to the Chambers' house, where Mr and Mrs Chambers had dressed up for an evening out.

'I was reading in the *Post* about someone that's defamed the Thomas Moore statue,' said Mr Chambers, squeezing his lapels like a barrister.

'Defaced, do you mean?'

'With pink paint.'

I was puzzled. 'Which Thomas Moore statue?' I asked.

Mr Chambers plainly thought I was slow. 'At the university. The Thomas Moore statue.'

I realised he meant the Henry Moore sculpture that stood on the main campus not far from the library. Some angry students had daubed it with poster paint as a sign of their seriousness. The grounds staff had to spend more than five minutes wiping it off with a rag.

'We go ballroom dancing on Monday,' said Mr Chambers, swerving suddenly into a new lane. 'That's why we're dressed in our refinery.'

It seemed to me that I couldn't last long at the Chambers' without being driven crazy. I felt I was in a different country, one with a similar language but a mysterious culture and no etiquette book.

After buying a bag of chips and eating them on my own in the silent dining room I went up to the bedroom. Net curtains covered the window and a decorative fan was arranged behind a print of orange horses galloping through the surf. Like the famous dolly–zoom shot in Hitchcock's *Vertigo* the room seemed to be changing perspective in a way that was hard to understand. It was very warm, and I couldn't turn down the radiator. I noticed a ringing in my ears.

Things seemed to have gone wrong somewhere. I was a facsimile of myself. An impostor. I was maintaining an exhausting camouflage, a mask. There was a veil between me and everyone else. The real me was hidden. Always had been hidden. Few spoke to me and though I made some bungled attempts to start up conversations, they petered out. I felt completely alone.

I decided to go out. Going out was better. I took a bus into town and walked along the main road towards the river. It was pelting down and the streetlamps were reflected in the varnished road, the spiderwebs heavy with rain. I reached a squat brown-and-cream church bleached at intervals by the headlights of passing cars. On the board was a notice: 'SOMETHING IS MISSING FROM THIS CH__CH: U. R.' Above this it said, 'Church of St Jude, Patron for the Hopeless and the Despaired'. I tried the door but unsurprisingly it was locked.

I wandered back into the street, which was shin-deep in the fallen leaves of the September plane trees. In the gutter lay the body of a ginger tomcat, eyes open, a thread of blood darkening the pavement beside his mouth. Hit by a car, I suppose. I walked past an empty café, past a door with a sign reading 'Dom Polski' and past a long industrial building with hundreds of chamber pots stacked in the window. Mock-antiques for export to the USA I imagined.

I went and sat in a huge ugly pub called the Janus. I had a pint of beer that made me shudder and watched the minutes tick slowly away. Everything in the pub was big: the tables, the pattern on the carpet, the noise coming out of the jukebox. It was a hall of mirrors.

Being a university town the usual uncouth toilet graffiti was augmented by more erudite benefactions. Over the toilet roll holder in the cubicle some wag had put: 'Sociology degrees. Help yourself.' Above this was neatly written: 'He was oppressed, and he was afflicted, yet he opened not his mouth!' Beside this it just said, 'BUM'.

I could see the past with knifelike sharpness, but not the future. I wished I could feel happy or excited about something. I went to the telephone box in the vestibule, where I tried to ring Jon back home. There was no answer. A couple in the corner seemed to be talking about me so I left the pub and boarded a juddering bus back to the house, letting myself in with the key on the Lions Club key ring that Mrs Chambers had given me. It was just gone nine o'clock. I got into bed and fell asleep to the sound of a buzzing streetlamp.

★

I wasn't sure how long I had been awake, but a hard moon was silhouetting the weft of the curtains. I'd been having a nightmare, which had faded, leaving me with only the horrible feeling attached to it. I got up and looked into the blue deserted road.

Solitude had been my refuge from loneliness, which, it seemed, came most when I was with other people. But the strain of getting through each self-punishing hour had exhausted me. I had imploded. I was down a black hole, thinking only of myself, because I had to survive. I was swimming in armour.

The abrupt changes of the past few days, the new town, the new routines, the incessant new information, the endless decisions and demands, the overstimulation, and the flubbed social overtures were all too much. I burst into tears.

My psyche, which had been frail for some time, was starting to come apart in my hands. Rooms were not really shrinking in on me: I was losing touch with reality.

In the morning, through a towering effort, I made it into the university. There were a few days left of self-regulated freedom before the official start of the academic year the following Monday. I had reached a turning point, the point at which relief from the suffering had become the vital thing. What I did that day is lost to me but at some moment I decided to stop, or anyway did stop, taking my insulin. The consequences of this I understood.

Autistic people die significantly younger than members of the typical population. At the more severe end of the continuum, it is epilepsy that does it. At the Asperger's end — where they are twice as likely as people in general to die young — it is suicide. This increased suicide risk is not a minor one: Aspergers are nine times more likely to deliberately kill themselves than non-autistic people. To say I had resolved to end my life is, though, not exactly right. Though it is silliness to live when to live is torment, all I really wanted was for the intolerable pain to stop. Just draw down the curtain and make it stop.

My decline was steady. I became extravagantly thirsty, exhausted. I sat on my bed or wandered confused around the campus. I stumbled and tripped. My eyes became blurred. I lost weight. I gasped for breath. Jagged pains cramped my back. My body was eating itself; shutting down. There was nobody to notice.

One evening in my bedroom at the Chambers' I found myself bent double, groaning in anguish. I staggered into the hallway and collapsed. This was it. Mrs Chambers called an ambulance. I faded to black.

★

I faded in again. There was a twisted square of light on the bright wall opposite. This was not a room I recognised. I was under a white sheet. Much of the furniture was white. A brisk nurse came in. This was some sort of hospital.

'Back with us, then? Let's sit you up. The doctor will be coming to see you in a minute.'

A pleasant breeze drifted through the window and I could hear a blackbird singing. The door opened and in glided a confident man in his forties, wearing a grey double-breasted jacket. His hair was polished and there was about him an ambience of kindliness, humour, and aftershave.

'I'm Doctor Alexander,' he said. 'How are you feeling?'

I made a face.

'You're in the university medical centre. Your blood glucose is off the radar and your body is consuming its own muscle. What we're going to do is get your insulin sorted out and once your numbers start coming down we'll slowly try to get some weight back on you. We'll monitor you for a bit. Doing things too quickly — that's how you make mistakes.'

I nodded.

'Anything you need? Anyone you'd like to talk to?'

I shook my head.

Dr Alexander was the first person since I had arrived at the university to pay close attention to me, to say something kind.

They had been feeding me water enriched with salt and glucose and now they wanted me to eat. But I had no appetite and was turning away food. One day I caught sight of my face in the mirror. It was cadaverous. When my parents came to visit they looked terrified. The nurses tried preparing all kinds of stuff for me but the taste of a piece of melon — which they sent out for after I had said I might manage it — was so strong that I was unable to swallow it. The brisk nurse lost her temper, which frightened me so much that I forced myself to chew a corner of dry toast and gradually I was able to build up my appetite again.

After I had put on a bit of weight she came in one evening.

'I'm sorry I barked at you,' she said, 'but we were so worried. We thought you might ...'

'What? Die?'

'Let's get these pillows sorted out a bit,' she said, plumping them with unnecessary force.

When Dr Alexander discharged me two weeks later I was still very thin. He gave me a penetrating look. He realised, I think, that there was more to this than met the eye. 'I never forget my diabetic patients,' he said, writing his name and number on a slip of paper and pushing it across to me. 'Ring me up any time you need to.'

Having missed the first couple of weeks in the art department, I approached Austin Randall to explain my absence. He seemed not to be listening and kept looking over my shoulder. His understanding of his pastoral role was, I felt, poor.

I went to my space to arrange my paints and brushes. Partitions separated me from a girl called Lucile on one side and I forget who on the other.

'I owe you a tube of chrome yellow,' said a voice. It belonged to a young man with a thick orange moustache who was wiping a brush in a space on the other side of the room.

'I'm going for a coffee,' he said. 'Fancy one?'

He peeled off his overalls and we strolled along the cloister. I caught sight of Fleeta Swit ambling across the lawn, a length of toilet paper flapping from her shoe. On the fascia of a large shed-like construction in an area behind one of the buildings the hand-painted word 'Refectory' announced its purpose. My new acquaintance ordered coffee, I asked for tea, and we crossed the creaking floor to one of the tables.

'I'm Anthony White,' he said.

'Hello,' I said. My portcullis was still down.

Anthony was a couple of years older than me, he liked football, which made my heart sink, but he also knew a great deal about the history of modern painting, Marvel comics, and black-and-white B-movies. He was dressed in a natty thirties tie and cavalry twill trousers as if for the role of a passerby in a film about plucky Londoners carrying on regardless as their houses are blitzed around them.

'We thought you'd chucked yourself in the river,' said Anthony.

'Bit under the weather,' I said. 'Been banged up in the medical centre.'

'I sneaked a tube of chrome yellow out of your box,' he said.

'Keep it,' I said.

'You're the focus of quite a bit of gossip. You've scared half of them stiff. You look so haughty.'

I was astonished. This was the first time I had heard myself described in this way, but it wouldn't be the last. My social dread was being mistaken for disdain. I thought I had been invisible but it wasn't other people who were being standoffish, it was, apparently, me.

I spoke to Anthony every day for the next four years and I have known him now for four decades. He sends me beautifully painted birthday cards, and the other day an invitation to his sixtieth birthday dropped onto the mat. Though we meet only occasionally we pick up right where we left off. Much of life hangs on the throw of the dice and if Anthony had not run out of chrome yellow that day it is possible we would never have become friends.

In the evening, he invited me up for dinner at his hall of residence on the main campus. Starley Hall was a three-storey brickwork enormity so ugly it made you laugh. Named after a dead vice chancellor, it resembled a 1960s barracks: four sheer walls enclosing a square of prison-like corridors overlooking a meagre lawn. It was the only single-sex hall in the university, and was, I learnt, favoured by rugby players. The clattering of studs down the passages was a constant background sound effect.

Anthony took me into the bar, where a banner announced: 'Freshers' Week 1978'. The date had been crudely done in black pen over a palimpsest of deletions going back years. I ordered two pints of beer and a packet of peanuts, which the barman pulled from a display card decorated with a lady in a cowboy hat and very short shorts. We carried our food over to a bench, where we sat down and surveyed the room.

Tongue-and-groove pine slats clad the walls and a pair of self-closing ship's kitchen doors led into a dining room that gave off a perfume of meat pie and disinfectant. The bar's ceiling was pocked with gobbets of dried Blu Tack, drawing pins, and bits of Christmas tinsel. A handful of pink-faced boys, one with a haircut like an erect horse's mane, were chatting and laughing beside a coin-operated telephone.

'We're having curry,' said Anthony.

'Who's "we"?' I asked warily.

'Rick, me, and a chap called Bill Bradshaw. You'll like him, he's unusual.'

Dr Alexander had instructed me to stuff in the calories, and wanting very much not to be alone I agreed to join Anthony and the others for curry. We walked up the corridor to Bill Bradshaw's kitchen area, which was, so it was said, the liveliest in the hall, and the place to be seen.

A fug of cigarette smoke hung in the air and Rick, who like us was a first year art student, was preparing to go round to the curry house. I had seen him chatting to four girls that morning, flicking his golden hair over his shoulder with studied nonchalance. Anthony introduced us and Rick told me he had once smashed a guitar over the head of a drummer who he found having sexual intercourse with his girlfriend. 'You hit the wrong person there,' I said.

'Tom's joining us for curry,' said Anthony.

'What do you want?' asked Rick, waving a menu at me.

'He'll have the same as me!' bellowed a reverberant voice. Down the corridor buzzed a barrel-chested man in an electric wheelchair, which he was directing with his toe. His legs were essentially thighs with feet on the end and he seemed to have no arms. He was the source of the cigarette smoke.

'Shake hands, newcomer,' he said, proffering his bare right foot by lifting it off the special tray he had on the front of his chair. This was Bill Bradshaw, a man who was to become one of my closest friends. I took his foot awkwardly and shook it. Bill bent forward and replaced between his first and second toes the cigarette he had been sucking.

'Ever eaten a phaal?' he asked, coughing through a cloud of smoke.

'What is it?' I asked.

'It's the hottest fucking curry ever.'

'Hotter than vindaloo?'

'Suck it and see,' said Bill.

I felt that a challenge had been issued. Though anxious by

nature, and cautious by principle, there is a contradictory risk-taking element to my character. 'All right,' I said.

'Get extra beer!' Bill shouted after Rick. A lot of university life so far seemed to involve drink.

There was a pregnant pause. I didn't see how I could not refer to Bill's unusual bodily construction without it becoming something, if left, that was forever too late to mention.

'If you don't mind my asking,' I said, 'what in God's name happened to you?' There was a guffaw followed by rather a lot of coughing.

'Bluntness gets points,' said Bill. 'It's a congenital condition, Tom. It's called, "phocomelia". It's not thalidomide. Let's open those cans.'

Bill told me he was in the second year of a linguistics degree, and said he was related to the Bradshaws, of *Bradshaw's Railway Timetable* fame, which I knew about from its mention in the Sherlock Holmes stories.

Bill's beer-drinking technique was intriguing. He would bend forward, grip the rim of the pint glass with his teeth, and lift it off his tray before tilting it back to swallow a mouthful.

When the curries arrived, a semicircle was formed around Bill and me. We opened our foil containers, the contents of which were black as the sea. I peered into the depths. Everything solid seemed to have been dissolved. Pouring the treacly phaal over the rice, I gave it a nervous sniff. The miasma made me splutter.

'Ah, the mystic Orient,' said Bill. 'Well, here goes.'

Gripping his fork between his toes he bent double, inserted a mouthful of curry, and sat up again, chewing vigorously.

I took my first, deliberately small, mouthful and chewed it like a debutante. It was certainly spicy, but nothing special. I took another, more generous, forkful and became aware of a creeping conflagration beginning at the back of my throat but spreading forwards until my head was engulfed. Tears came to my eyes and I started to cough. Rick passed me a can of beer. 'Alcohol dissolves it,' he said urgently. Water only makes it worse.'

Bill was clearly suffering too. Rivulets of sweat were rolling down his temples into his bushy beard.

'Well?' he asked, through a mouthful of food.

Bravado seemed the best plan. 'It's a bit warm,' I said. 'I'll give you that.'

The others finished their curries and tipped their plates into the sink. Then they sat down to watch us. Breaths were held.

We ended the ordeal pretty much together and though my gorge was ablaze I became conscious of a feeling of anaesthetic calm. 'Endorphins,' said Bill. I think it was the first time I had heard the word. We wiped our foreheads and Bill lit a cigarette. I had passed the test.

I began spending more and more time at Starley Hall with Anthony and Bill. At the end of the first term Mr and Mrs Chambers decided that accommodating students, or, at least, accommodating *me*, was perhaps not what they were cut out for, and they asked me to leave. So, at Anthony's nudging, I took over the place of a student who had just moved out of Starley. It was a warm, decent-sized ground-floor room with a regular cleaning lady, a single bed, bookshelves, and a window onto the shrivelled quad.

Much of the first year in the art department was spent suffering the indignities of the daft exercises that we were continually set. I wanted to draw things I could see but was told that this was 'mere illustration'. I felt like Josef K. accused of some mysterious crime, without having done anything wrong. Why this loathing for the

human drive to record what we see? I wondered. To me, cave paintings, Rembrandt, and Rothko were part of the same story.

Instead of matter-of-factly going along with things I took it
all too much to heart. If Miss Legge could have seen me now she
would have railed at me again for having turned up my nose at the
Central School. The trouble with advice is that you cannot tell the
good from the bad until it's too late.

One student who took the whole thing in his stride was Charley
Lindsay, a boozy and charming young fellow who knew how the
system worked and how to work it. He did almost nothing for
four years because he was permanently propping up the bar in the
Beehive or the Turk's Head. Everybody including the teaching staff
liked Charley, even though they barely saw him outside the pub.
One evening, full of beer, he fell downstairs holding a knife and cut
his little finger tendon, which they replaced with a bit of toe.

'If they ask if I've had my bowels open,' said Charley when I
saw him in hospital, 'I always say yes.'

'Why?' I asked.

'Tell people what they want to hear; it makes life easier.'

I was impressed by this worldliness but repelled by the dishonesty. Someone later whispered that Charley Lindsay was actually
Charles Lloyd-Lindsay, who had learned at nanny's knee how to
glide along on life's gondola while some other poor fool pushed
with the stick. Not for Charlie the bleak single-sex Starley Hall.
The rumour was that he, like fellow students who had been to
public school or who were otherwise perceived to be of good stock,
had got himself put up in Christ Church Hall, a building of Tudor
pretensions, endowed with crenellated turrets and stone archways.
Such shameless social engineering, if that's what it was, struck me as
squalid. Others, less moralistic, just shrugged.

Every art student had to take art history as a subsidiary first-year subject. Anthony and I had agreed that one year of art history would be a doddle for most of us painters, and so it proved. We did not mingle with the art historians, none of whom seemed particularly interested in painting, or aesthetics, or being painters themselves. They were like eunuchs in the harem: they knew how it was done; they saw it done every day; but they were unable to do it themselves.

The subject of art almost never came up in art history lectures. There was instead a zeal for dates, schools of painting, the politics of the time, who had known whom, who had done what to whom, and, most absurdly, what paintings were called. The only thing I remember of the art history professor was that, while working in the beautiful art library one Sunday, he tripped on a Turkish rug and went hands-first through the glass doors of a bookcase. Microsurgeons at the nearby hospital had their work cut out.

I recall only one art history lecturer with any clarity, a softly spoken young Scotsman with degrees in law, philosophy, and modern languages from a number of distinguished British and French universities, as well as one in art history from the Courtauld Institute of Art, where the spy Anthony Blunt had admired his oomph. Somebody said, 'That man is chair material,' which puzzled me.

The man's name was Neil MacGregor and he went on to run the National Gallery and the British Museum. Though I have forgotten everything he told us about painting, sculpture, and architecture, I do remember that during one of his talks some people were nattering. 'Will you please shut up at the back!' he said. Though not good enough, perhaps, for a book of quotations, this did stick in my mind.

As well as art history, all undergraduates had to pass a first-year exam in a third subject, one of their own choosing. I plumped for philosophy, imagining stimulating tutorials in which we would be thrashing out tricky problems such as 'What is beauty?' or 'How ought one to behave?' or 'Does it make any sense to talk about the "meaning" of life?' As it turned out, we were just told to read a lot of old books and attend tedious lectures. The only chance to discuss ideas came in tutorials during which everyone spoke in a pre-agreed code that was gobbledegook to me. They used terms like *naturalistic fallacy* and *secundum quid*, which sounded like the final part of a two-part payment.

The only time I scored a point in philosophy was when I declined an invitation to agree that atoms were real. 'Aha!' said the tutor, 'Another Wittgenstein.' As a young man, Ludwig Wittgenstein, one of the most influential philosophers of the twentieth century, had famously annoyed Bertrand Russell by refusing to accept that there was not a rhinoceros in the room.

Like Hans Asperger, Ludwig Wittgenstein (1889–1951) was born in Vienna, the youngest of nine children. His father was described as a harsh perfectionist, lacking in empathy. His mother was characterised as anxious. He was almost certainly autistic.

As a boy, Ludwig was fascinated by machinery and was so technically adept that by the age of ten he was able to make a working model of a sewing machine out of bits of wire and wood.

The family was musically educated; his father was a good violinist, and his brother became a celebrated concert pianist, who continued playing even after he lost an arm. Ludwig himself had absolute pitch and could whistle lengthy and intricate tunes. He played the clarinet and also composed.

He had a superb sense of proportion and later in life he designed a house for his sister Margaret, paying very close attention to every detail: drawing each window, door, lock, and radiator with such care that they might have been precision instruments. It took him a year to design just the door handles. The radiators, another year. Nothing was unimportant.

Unsociable and strange, with mad staring eyes, Wittgenstein had very few friends throughout his life and found even simple social exchanges difficult. *The Times* reported his periods of 'extreme abnegation and retirement', likening him to, 'a religious hermit of the contemplative type'.

He studied aeronautical engineering and later became a mechanical engineer. At other times he was a schoolmaster and a gardener for a monastery, where he inquired about becoming a monk. Engineering, gardening, and philosophy are all systems-based occupations attractive to the autistic mind. They demand, like the routines of the monk, little in the way of sociability.

In Christopher Sykes' BBC film *A Wonderful Life* (1989), the wife of Wittgenstein's doctor, with whom he was staying at the time of his death, said that Ludwig refused to shake hands, and, 'seemed as oblivious as if he was walking through us ... Normally he sat at breakfast facing a window, not speaking to anyone ... He was just the man in the corner.'

He suffered from terrific loneliness, and depression was his constant companion, as it had been for three of his brothers, who killed themselves. He too continually thought of suicide. 'My day passes,' he said, 'between logic, whistling, going for walks, and being depressed.'

Sulky, snappish, sensitive, and nervous, he was attuned to any change in mood, or the tiniest slight. In spite of this personal touchiness he could himself be very offensive. The physicist and mathematician Freeman Dyson at first took exception to being on the receiving end of his rudeness, but later made allowances: 'He was a tortured soul,' he said, 'living a lonely life among strangers …' Philosopher Anthony Quinton described him as 'an extremely isolated figure, perhaps locked up mainly in his own thoughts'.

Like many autistics, Wittgenstein found solace in nature: sailing, gardening, walking, and observing the natural world. Among his other interests were pulpy detective stories, which he loved. He also visited the cinema, where he insisted on sitting in the front row so that there was nothing in his field of vision but the screen.

Ludwig Wittgenstein is generally agreed to have been the most original philosopher of modern times, coming up with two entirely new, though incompatible, philosophies — one early in his philosophic life, the other late. These dealt with language, a frequent preoccupation of autistics. His special concern was with trying to work out how it is that language represents the world. Though his two different approaches became highly influential, he had, by the end of his life, disowned them both, stating that it was impossible to put into words anything that really mattered.

His writing was as distant and aloof as his personal behaviour. But despite his obsession with being intellectually 'well scrubbed' and his immensely fastidious insistence on precision and discipline, his gnomic *Tractatus Logico-Philosophicus* was obscure even to philosophers used to opacity. To the ordinary person it is about as much use as a chocolate teapot. When his English translator asked him what he had meant by certain things he either said he had forgotten or that he couldn't understand how he could have been such a fool as to write what it looked as though he might have meant. How much use is this sort of thing?

The otherworldliness of much philosophy and the abstract

peculiarity of its language started to annoy me, and as time passed I found myself drawn instead to science. Using scientific method you could make concrete predictions based on reliable underlying laws; science was testable, and it was less highfalutin. How I got through a whole year of philosophy beats me.

★

Spring followed winter and, as the wisteria's heavy perfume wafted across the campus, posters appeared asking for writers for the end-of-year review. I went along to a meeting and was overawed by the sophistication of some of the students there. Most were two or three years older than me, which seems an important difference at that age. Two of them — Andy and Jimmy — were doctoral students approaching their thirties. They seemed impossibly mature and wise. To my delighted amazement I recognised that much of the show's writing, produced mainly by Andy and Jimmy, was distinctly superior. How wonderful to find some people who really knew what they were doing. Of course it wasn't exclusively top notch: after becoming irritated in early rehearsals by the constant reference to a kangaroo as a mammal I approached Andy, who was directing. 'That should be "marsupial",' I said. 'It's more precise and it's a funnier word in context.'

'See what you can do with this,' he said, stuffing a crumpled sketch into my hand, making me suddenly an accidental script doctor. I remember suggesting a few improvements, including some language jokes with a German lady at a bus stop and a bit of business with cucumbers in a bicycle basket. Andy chuckled but I was sure he would soon find me out as the impostor I was.

At the end of the year I somehow passed my exams and got

myself a job for the long vacation in a town down the river with a pretty suspension bridge. In the high street was a hotel and it was here that I was to be employed as barman and factotum.

Charley told me he had landed a job as a whisky deliveryman. Any breakages, he was warned, and he must return the bottle's unbroken cap seal. 'What I do,' he said, 'is turn the bottle upsidedown and hit it below the label with a steel ruler. The bottom flies off and you can then drink the Scotch and return the seal intact.' I was shocked.

Reporting for my hotel job on the first day, I met the boss, an Italian who combed the remaining six strands of his hair over his shining scalp. He introduced me to a few of my new colleagues including a pretty young waitress from Wolverhampton and a chef called Mike: cynic, lothario, and wit. Mike pointed to the kitchen cookers, which were mounted on casters and stood in huge stainless-steel trays that caught the dripping fat, custard, and fallen scraps of food. 'A company came to clean those trays recently,' he told me. 'They pulled out the cookers and underneath was a gigantic carpet of pus.' It was a vivid picture he painted.

Gerry the washer-upper was scrubbing an oven tray and wanted to tell me about his favourite subject — his time in the Far East after the war.

'What do you remember best?' I asked, hoping for some historical colour.

'Those Japanese girls,' he said. 'They'll do *anything*.' I noticed a blob of ash drop from his cigarette onto a tray of tomato salad.

There were several bars in the hotel and I was kept busy, learning on the job. I was very anxious at the beginning, partly because of my inability to chat with customers, and partly because of my severe problem with numbers, which made it difficult to work out prices fast, especially when customers were three deep at the bar, all shouting and waving pound notes. Out of desperation I came up with my own method: calculating the pounds first and adding the pennies afterwards. This resulted in weird mental sums that went, 'One pound forty-four, plus three pounds twenty-eight, that's four pounds sixty-twelve.' But it worked for me.

The assistant manager was a compact fellow of about my age, whose mission was to become a silver-service waiter. He was bright and ambitious but prematurely world-weary having got his girlfriend pregnant while still at school. Trapped in a curdled marriage he found his job a release from the limbo of dirty nappies and tired harangues. At the end of my first shift, which flew past, he came to help me with the mountain of glasses.

'Do you want to wash or dry?' he asked.

'I'll die,' I said, which kept him laughing for several weeks.

I was being put up in the staff lodgings, where I briefly shared a room with a Parisian student who wore red silk underpants to bed. Other members of this transitory menagerie were a Portuguese chef and his dishwashing wife. In a hutch at the end of the scrappy garden the chef kept rabbits that he fussed over like a dowager. One day I saw him in tears after he had broken the neck of one and cooked it for his dinner. His wife explained in stumbling English that this was the purpose of these animals, but that it made him cry every time.

One sultry evening after the clamour had died down I was tidying the bottles behind the bar, a repetitive classification job ideal for the systemising mind. The pretty Wolverhampton waitress, whose name was Soraya, came over. She was engaged to another hotel employee, a prognathic clod with wide shoulders.

'Would you like to go out for a meal?' she asked without preamble. I was immediately alert.

'How do you mean?' I said.

'Brett's going to a party and he won't take me,' she said.

'Are you sure that's wise?'

'Look, it's just food. Nothing else.'

Having lived like a monk for too long, the promise of female company sounded like just what the doctor ordered, so I agreed. A more experienced person might have warned me that this was not a good idea.

We were to meet in a local restaurant so I showered and ran a comb through my hair and through the highly unfashionable handlebar moustache that I was beginning to cultivate. I walked the short distance to the place. Soraya had got there before me.

'Hello,' I said. 'What would you like to drink?'

'I've got butterflies,' she said.

At this moment warning sirens should have gone off, but instead of thanking her for a delightful evening and going straight home I went to the bar.

During dinner I was discretion itself. Afterwards she wanted to walk along the river but halfway over the bridge she stopped me.

'Tom,' she said.

'What?'

'Are you gay?'

'No,' I said. 'Why do you ask?'

'Because you're the only man I've ever met who doesn't try it on all the time.'

'But you're engaged,' I said. 'And anyway that is not a respectful way to behave.' I was starting to sound like the Most Reverend Donald Coggan.

'I've never met anyone like you,' said Soraya, suddenly clasping my hand and intertwining her fingers with mine. Full of beer and also wine I did not dissuade her.

'Let's go down here,' I said, indicating a secluded spot on the riverbank. She stiffened immediately.

'No,' she said. 'I know what men are like. You all want the same thing.' I got the feeling that she had been hanging around with the wrong sort of men.

'We'll just sit on the bench,' I said. I led her down and we sat beside each other listening to the lapping water. We discussed what she had seen on the television, why southerners pronounced 'jug' 'jag' instead of 'joog', and, less trivially, her unhappy life at home in the West Midlands, where all men wanted the same thing.

I looked up into the crisp sky. I could see several constellations, and recalled my boyhood interest in astronomy. I squeezed Soraya's arm and pointed out Cassiopeia. I watched the soft light on her upturned nose as she inspected the constellation's giant W for the first time in her life. She was a remarkably pretty, intelligent girl who seemed horribly ill informed about almost everything.

A church carillon sounded the quarters. She stopped and looked steadily into my eyes. Then she let go of my fingers and very deliberately put her palm into my lap. Catalysed by the alcohol pumping through my temples, desire erupted and I roughly took hold of her. She moaned luxuriantly.

Nemesis follows hubris and next morning the boyfriend demanded to interrogate me in the bar. A background tape was playing a quiet medley of hits, and to the accompaniment of an ersatz Nancy Sinatra singing a soundalike version of *These Boots Are Made for Walkin'* I delivered in my defence a series of statements that, though strictly true, were non-incriminating. My bland account of a dullish evening somehow persuaded the boyfriend that I hadn't been a-messin' where I shouldn't've been a-messin' and that his girlfriend's late arrival home minus certain articles of clothing was innocuous. Thus I avoided being punched. I convinced myself that my brain had been too subtle for his brawn, though I did wonder afterwards whether Soraya hadn't just told him I was gay.

Though my stonewalling had been strictly truthful, I knew it had also been dishonest and this troubled me. I consoled myself that the preservation of my teeth had been a justifiable motive. I was also concerned that this oaf might take physical revenge on Soraya. And of course I was young. And of course I had not been the one pushing it. And of course I had been drunk. This is called 'rationalisation'.

I wonder what pretty little Soraya is doing today. She must be sixty. Has she retained her naive poise, or ballooned out, lost teeth, and been shunned by the men who once all wanted the same thing but no longer want it, at least not from her?

★

The leaves were trembling along the river and the holiday was coming to an end. There was a new assistant manager who was annoying everyone by poncing about smoking Balkan Sobranie cigarettes through a holder. Custom was slackening off and summer staff were leaving the hotel. Soraya and her fiancé had gone to Weston-super-Mare and Mike the chef thought he might join the army.

On my last day I knocked off early and went to look round the church that had chimed the quarters as I sat beside Soraya that night. It was a Victorian Gothic number with a skinny stone spire and chequered flushwork. As I walked into the cool interior the door swung shut with a boom. Pews were ranked among the great yellow arches, and dusty standards hung from the walls. I sat down under a discreet loudspeaker and thought about Katy. She was somewhere now, doing something. I could draw a line from where I was sitting to wherever she was. We were physically connected. Everything was connected. I got on the train back to the university.

After ten weeks of dehydrated breakfast mushrooms and carousing rugby clubbers I had decided to move out of Starley Hall and was to spend the rest of my four years in a small but convenient bedsitting room in the town. The room was in the attic of an Edwardian house, my neighbours on the top landing being a giant black man who played eye-watering reggae that shook the rafters while he bellowed into a microphone, and a pale bearded Scotsman called Tim Scattergood who brought a different woman back to his flat each night. The walls were thin and when I wasn't being kept awake by the pounding music I was listening to the squeaking of Tim's springs and the grunts of his various lady friends. On the floor below me lived a strange man who wore kilts and cried himself to sleep.

During the second year we were left more to our own devices in the art department. I learned etching and also lithography, a technique unchanged since the eighteenth century. First you drew onto a smooth stone with a greasy pencil. Then you applied acid and gum arabic, which smelt of cat's pee when it went off. You then wet the stone and applied ink, which stuck only to the original greasy drawing. Finally you overlay a sheet of paper and put the stone to press. The magic moment came when you peeled back the paper to reveal your drawing, in reverse. The work I produced was heartily loathed by the teaching staff, and they let me know it.

I became vaguely friendly with a student called Diana. She had been to an expensive school in Highgate and was polished. I was talking to her one day about turps or something and jiggling my leg, as I like to do. 'Don't do that in my space, please Tom,' she said with a laugh. Diana's dad had bought her a house in town. The wallpaper was peeling and each door was sloppily painted in different colours, which unsettled me. Diana let out rooms to students, including Anthony, who, like me, had moved out of Starley Hall. One of her tenants smelt very strongly of antiseptic. She took me to his room. 'Have a look,' she said, pushing open the door with her elbow. Thousands of empty TCP bottles covered the floor and the bed. The smell was hard to describe.

Some of Diana's tenants were girls from the art department. Alice, the strawberry blonde who ignored me, had a room near the staircase and was often obliged to pass me as I sat talking to Anthony in the kitchen. After a while she began to nod grudgingly when she went in or out of her room. One day we were discussing the Sony Walkman, a newish battery-run gadget for listening to cassettes through earphones while you walked along. Was the plural 'Walkmen' or 'Walkmans'? I wondered. Alice didn't know. She smiled mysteriously.

Jon, my friend from school, had moved to London to study at the Slade. He was staying in a hall of residence near King's Cross, not far from the National Youth Theatre, where Michael Croft had looked me up and down in his office a few years before. King's Cross is now a sterile promontory of gentrification, craft beer, and *al fresco* dining. When Jon was there it was a lovely shithole of tarts and drunks.

I began travelling to London on a Friday evening and staying on Jon's floor over the weekend, a procedure I kept up over three years. I spent more than I could afford on a plaster bust of William Blake from the National Portrait Gallery. It stands on my bookcase today, next to an old box of Woodbine cigarettes. One day I stopped off in the Berkshire village of Cookham to visit the Stanley Spencer museum. Spencer, whose work I liked, was a peculiar painter and a peculiar man. Slovenly looking, he dressed in ludicrous hats and grubby looking formal jackets, frequently with his pyjamas underneath. In the rare interviews that I have seen he makes no eye contact whatever.

He had a strange, distant relationship with his two daughters, one of whom said that he, 'needed to be alone a great deal ... he had to go into himself and rummage around and walk about inside himself'. He was curiously naive, and, to everyone's dismay, married a lesbian freeloader who moved her partner into his house before taking him to the cleaners and evicting him.

Spencer had a series of narrowly focused unchanging interests, including painting, sex, and the Bible. He would traipse through the lanes of Cookham pushing an old pram full of paints and brushes, recording in abnormal detail every leaf and blade of grass. He was also a prolific writer of lists, which documented, among other things, every single plant he had included in his paintings.

At the time I didn't know that these peculiarities were autistic traits. All I knew was that Stanley Spencer reminded me very much of Bob Strange, the intense student who stuck cocktail sticks into cigars.

After my visit to Cookham I got back on the train to continue my trip to London. It was one of those clanking slam-door trains that used to call at all the halts and produce a lot of diesel smoke. In time we pulled up at a quiet station where an old man supporting himself on two sticks clambered aboard. As we took off I noticed that although he and I were the only occupants of the carriage he had chosen to sit on the seat across the aisle from me.

We had been jiggling along for a few minutes when I became aware that I was being watched. I peered furtively at the old man's reflection and he caught my eye. I looked him in the face.

'Is your name Thomas?' he asked quite suddenly.

Although I am not prone to supernatural woo-woo an eerie thrill ran through me. Being of a scientific bent I tried to work out what rational thing might explain the accuracy of his query: a wild guess? (improbable), an elaborate prank? (even less likely), or did the old fellow think he knew me? If so, how did he know my name and who could he possibly be?

I thought I might have some identifying label hanging from my bag or coat, like a wartime evacuee, but I quickly decided against this. In any case, nobody called me Thomas except my parents.

Then it struck me that this serious-faced old chap might be my long-lost grandfather, the bigamist, who had abandoned his family, but kept in touch sporadically with my father, enough to know my name.

'Yes,' I said, 'that's right.'

He gave me a respectful nod. 'Thomas the cat,' he mused, looking kindly at me for a moment.

'Where do you live?'

I told him.

'Oh yes,' he said. 'A nice town. A nice place.' He smiled a rather wistful smile and turned slowly away to watch the sunny banks and trees passing by his window.

I sucked my teeth. Should I take things further or should I let sleeping dogs lie? Before I had come to a conclusion, we drew into a station, where he got off with his two sticks, as best he could. Slamming the door, he gave me a searching look through the glass before disappearing down the underpass. I saw him come up on another platform, where he stood inscrutably in his grey coat. The train sat for some time ticking over and I had half a mind to jump out and ask him some questions. But before I could act the whistle blew and we began grinding noisily out of the station.

As we chugged away towards London I felt pretty sure that I had been speaking to my grandfather. Had he recognised in my face the face of his own son? I wished I had taken the time to question him. There was so much we both could have said. He had been an engineer. Did he, I wonder, share the family's Asperger genes? Had he passed them on to my father, who passed them on to my brother and to me? Who knows what turn my life might have taken had I got off that train and spoken to him? He will be many years dead, that old man, but I often think of him that day, long ago and far away.

★

I went along to a meeting in the students' union of the group who were interested in starting a university radio station. It never got off the ground while I was there, though a portable tape recorder was acquired. I borrowed this one evening and took it along to a concert in town given by the American jazz guitarist Barney Kessel. With an audacity that I now find hard to credit I asked an usher if Kessel would be prepared to talk to somebody 'from the university radio station'. She went away and returned promptly to say I should go backstage in the interval.

When I went round I found that Kessel's relaxed onstage persona disguised the truly alarming intelligence and seriousness of the man. I had read about the techniques you needed for a good interview, and it was a good job I had prepared, because this was my first radio interview and Kessel had done a thousand of them. During the twenty-five minutes he generously gave me he absolutely kept me on my toes. Though I had jumped in the deep end I found that I enjoyed interviewing. It was a safe imitation of conversation, without any room for the social prattle I found so hard.

The next day there was a letter for me on the hallway table. I recognised the blue handwriting and was astonished. It was from Katy. I took it upstairs and read it through. It was a mildly friendly note telling me that she had started her studies in London and suggesting a meeting. I tried to fancy what the flame of a candle was like after the candle was blown out, for I could not remember ever having seen such a thing. I replied politely, accepting the proposed date and time. Then I went over to see Bill Bradshaw, who had moved into a wheelchair-friendly flat near some shops.

Nodding at a printed card on his tray, he made a suggestion.

'I've been invited to this thing in London. Fancy coming along as my official wheelchair pusher?'

I looked at the invitation. It was from a set-up run by Lord Snowdon, the recently divorced husband of Princess Margaret. The purpose of this organisation was to award grants to disabled students.

'You don't need a wheelchair pusher,' I said.

'It's going to be boring,' said Bill. 'I need a drinking companion.'

'Okay,' I said.

The awards event was taking place in a large private room at the South Bank complex and Bill was driving us in his crazy-looking adapted car. The sight of him sailing along, steering with his foot, could give you pause for thought, since he was as carefree a driver as he was an eater, drinker, and smoker.

'This is the Seven Bends of Death,' he shouted cheerfully as we shot round a hairpin turn. He treated the speed limit as an advisory minimum, and, as we hurtled towards our destination, I held on to anything stable.

After a near miss on Hyde Park Corner, Bill parked without

incident. When we got to the door we were ushered into a long room with blond wood and soft carpeting, issued with tea in china cups, and encouraged to mingle.

I was frozen with anxiety at the number of self-assured men, and women chuckling ambassador's-wife chuckles. Everyone was kitted out in sharp lounge suits or stylish dresses, whether or not blessed with a full complement of limbs. Bill and I were quite a contrast to other guests. My hair was unfashionably long at the time and there was paint residue and printer's ink on my hands. I probably seemed terse and offhand. Bill rarely dressed smartly and didn't own a suit. Hiring one was an expensive nuisance for him since few off-the-peg numbers were made for a four-foot-tall man with no arms.

'I don't go in for these "Cripple of the Year" contests,' he said.

'I notice you don't turn your nose up at the money,' I replied.

'Hello, hello,' said a voice. There, in a nimbus of cigar smoke, stood an extraordinary-looking pale-haired creature wearing a loud tracksuit. It was the children's television personality Jimmy Savile, widely esteemed for his charitable money-raising work. Bill was not to live long enough to witness Savile's saintly reputation being shattered by the discovery, decades later, of a fifty-year history of reported sex attacks on defenceless children.

'Traffic's terrible!' said Savile, through nicotine-yellow teeth. But before either of us could think of a sufficiently flavourless reply he spotted a teenage girl in a wheelchair and turned on his heel. I cannot say that he gave me the creeps exactly, but he did seem excessively self-interested, and his cigar-breath was unforgettably foul.

After the awards, a lady who was trying to arrange a group photograph beckoned Bill over. 'Picture then pub,' said Bill under his breath, pressing his wheelchair button and moving off into the photographer's bubble. As I waited, staring down at my scuffed shoes, I became aware of a man standing with his back to me. He had on a superbly cut grey suit and was smoking savagely. Another crisply dressed man with spectacles arrived at his side and leant forward discreetly. 'You have to be in the picture,' he said.

The smoking man shook his head.

'You must,' said Spectacles-man, pressing his lips together.

Smoking-man gave his head another shake: more emphatic this time. I searched my memory for anything similar that might explain what was happening. Was this man friendly? Was he dangerous? While maintaining the bearing of slightly sinister servant, he seemed to be in command of the smoking man. He struck me as the sort of creature who would not hesitate to push home the last inch of steel.

The smoking man turned resignedly, looking around for something. I recognised him at once as Lord Snowdon. He extended his arm. 'Hold this,' he said unsmilingly, handing over the rump of a cigarette that had been smoked to within an inch of its life. A chunk of ash hung on fiercely to a slender relict of unburnt tobacco. Any normal person would have stubbed the thing out. I took it and stood holding it hot end skywards as Snowdon moved into the group for the snap. To him I was nothing more than a human ashtray but I took no offence. People have reasons for the way they behave, and anyway the observation was an interesting one.

When the snapping was done Snowdon returned, plucked the stub from my grip without a word, and sucked it, like one of Bob Strange's cigars, into oblivion. I noticed as he did so that his hands trembled. I had the feeling he needed a drink.

'Let's get out of here,' said Bill.

We went to a vast black pub I knew under the railway arches near Waterloo station. It was dark and smelled deliciously of soot and dripping beer. Every time a train passed overhead the whole place rumbled, and glasses rattled against the tabletops.

'Are you okay?' said Bill, gripping his glass between his teeth. 'You seemed rather quiet in there, and you were a bit rude to that lady with the pearls.' I tried to explain, but I didn't understand. Why my permanent lover's quarrel with the world? Why could I not feel cheerful along with everyone else? We drove home fast but quietly.

Despite my continuing low mood, I was somehow still able to laugh. I read *Prick Up Your Ears*, John Lahr's biography of playwright Joe Orton, who used to send spoof letters to pompous officials under the name Edna Welthorpe (Mrs). On Valentine's Day 1967 Welthorpe wrote to the manager of the Ritz Hotel in London asking whether he had discovered her brown Morocco handbag, which contained, 'a few loose coins, a Boots folder with snapshots of members of my family, and a pair of gloves made of some hairy material'. On another occasion, she wrote to the manufacturers of a pie filling objecting to the inclusion of, '"EDIBLE STARCH" and "LOCUST BEAN GUM" ... My stomach really turned at what I saw when I opened the tin'. The way Orton used language made me laugh out loud. I wanted to write my own spoof letters.

It was a tremendous help to me that alcohol was a central pillar of student social life. After a pint or two, I always felt more at ease, more able to join in. It's not that drinking made me feel good so much as that it made me feel less bad. I am not a social drinker but neither do I drink alone at home. I like to be in a pub, where I sit in a corner in the company of strangers, watching. Luckily there were several wonderful pubs near the art department, one for every mood. There was the Turk's Head, where the landlady put lemon zest in the chicken sandwiches, the snug Beehive, and the Fisherman's Cottage on the canal, with fresh sawdust on the floor every day.

The inability to join in has always been the essence of my problem. So often, at school, at parties, at work, I was faced with other people's insistence that I join in with something thoroughly disagreeable. This expectation, I learnt recently, is known by human resources people as 'FIFO', standing for 'Fit In or Fuck Off', a charming philosophy that results in many Aspergers being socially shunned, excluded from work, and failed at school.

I found parties terribly difficult, but, wanting to fit in, I used to go along. Usually it was a disaster. Once or twice, to my dismay, someone offered me a marihuana cigarette, which I refused, before getting up and going home. My attitude to sex, drugs, and rock'n'roll was that I was all for the first but firmly against the second and third.

This was not Puritanism: it was, in the case of rock music, that I found the sound physically painful and emotionally upsetting. I cannot cope with so much noise and aggression in so distilled a compound. As for illegal drugs, my antipathy to them is that, being illegal, they ought not to be taken. Laws ought to be obeyed. I feel this very strongly. My attitude is, actually, that ordinary cannabis could probably be decriminalised, since it may well be less physically harmful than the very harmful legal drugs tobacco and alcohol. If it were made legal, however, I should object to it on two grounds. First: exclusivity. To someone who does not wish to smoke it, a shared marihuana cigarette is highly antisocial, a shibboleth that pushes him further out than before. Second: hygiene. Putting something in my mouth that has been in somebody else's mouth has always disgusted me. The marihuana cigarette is thus as nauseating as the communion cup of my boyhood, slathered with other people's spittle and crawling with faecal coliforms and who knows what else.

★

The swirling leaves from the plane trees gave way to feathers of frost on the inside of my bedsit window. One bitterly cold morning I awoke to ice on the surface of my blankets. Later my water pipe burst while I was out, flooding the flat downstairs.

I had arranged to visit Katy at her hall of residence in London. I was, of course, on time.

I rang the bell and she let me in.

I gave her some small present.

She thanked me.

I asked about her English course.

She told me about it. Did I want a cup of tea?

Yes please.

Should we go for a walk around the area?

Okay.

What time was my train home?

I was flexible.

Would I like to go to the pub?

Yes, okay.

So we went to the pub and had a drink by the fire. And then some more. Her knee accidentally touched my knee. It was late. I walked her back.

Did I want to come in before catching my train?

Okay.

She was sleepy. Did I mind if she lay on the bed?

How could I?

She seemed to have dozed off. I leant over her and she opened her eyes. They were like stars.

★

Many people look back on their time at university as one of the most enjoyable and freest periods of their life. For me it was the unhappiest time. As well as my difficulty with the enforced social expectations, I remained irked by the course and the quality of teaching, and indignant at the way I was being treated. Other students were also disaffected but understood how to change their circumstances. Both Bobs left, moving on to better places, and so we lost two interesting people. Lucile had a word with her uncle, who she said had connections with the Ruskin school, and she moved to Oxford. A new student named Harry Samson, who was in the year below me, made an official complaint to the professor. Before he knew what was happening he had been summoned for a grilling by the sub-dean. Coming back with his tail between his legs he told me that he too would be leaving.

One day a tutor berated me in front of the group: 'You are so uptight!' he scolded. 'Is there something wrong with you? You should get pissed! You're not an artist.' Being publicly ridiculed in this unkind way is not helpful to Aspergers — or anyone.

The autistic writer and television presenter Chris Packham has said that at university he was, 'confused … inordinately angry … absolutely raging.' I identify with this remark. My indignation had always been righteous and now it became focused. I composed a three-page letter of complaint, referring to the 'you should get pissed' incident. I addressed it to my tutor and copied it to the professor. Since Harry Samson had been levered out by deliberate use of the sub-dean I decided to give them a taste of their own medicine and copied it to him too.

The next morning I was drying a cup at my window when,

looking down from the eminence of my garret, I saw a tweedy middle-aged lady arrive on a bicycle. She got off holding a long white envelope, passed out of sight, and reappeared envelopeless before cycling off. I walked down to the hallway. Sure enough, there on the mat was a luxury envelope. On it, superbly typed, my name.

At the top of the enclosed heavily laid paper was the insignia of the vice chancellor. The thrust of his message was that he would very much like me to make an appointment, at my convenience, to discuss the letter I had posted the previous morning, which had been passed on to him by the sub-dean.

I was astonished by the speed of this response, by the careful hand delivery, and by the urgent politeness. Had I been more worldly I would have recognised the signs of a chief executive scared green that the business he was supposed to be running was conceivably about to be exposed in the press as one that was encouraging the teenagers in its care to 'get pissed'. But all this passed me by.

As requested, I made an appointment with the vice chancellor. He was genial, but at one moment his eyes narrowed: 'Three copies of your letter,' he mused. 'In long hand …'

The next day the professor, who generally had no contact with students, asked to see me. I walked into his sanctum. There were papers, a pipe rack, and a tin of coin tobacco. He was not smoking. Through gritted teeth he made me a subspecies of apology, at the end letting something slip: 'I find the vice chancellor a rather aggressive man,' he said.

'I found him charming,' I retorted.

I had them in the vice. One wrong move and they would get another rocket fired right up their department. But that was not my aim and I never mentioned the sorry business again. I had been intent only on doing whatever I could to overturn the injustice I felt. I was treated thereafter like a vibration-sensitive bomb in a shoebox. That is to say, their hostile movements became slower, craftier, more subtle.

The hounds of spring were on winter's traces and Katy had arranged to visit me. I tidied assiduously, washed linen, and bought flowers, which I put in a vase. This was nothing new. I often had flowers on the table and had always been fastidious. In this I was unlike many fellow students, the worst of whom posted his dirty laundry home to his mother, who returned it washed and ironed.

When Katy arrived something was wrong: she was distant. We went through the motions, but she seemed elsewhere. Afterwards I took her to the station. She said goodbye politely. Within a day or two I had a letter finally dismissing me.

Autistic people have great trouble accommodating change, and sudden romantic loss is withering change of the most permanent and painful kind, second only to bereavement by death. I struggled with the double-barrelled dispossession: taken away once, given back, taken away again. The course of true love never did run smooth, but what good had all this done?

It was my great fortune that there was a pressing distraction. The art department had organised a three-week trip to Paris, where we were to stay, all of us, in a rickety hotel near the Gare du Nord. I kept a callow diary of this expedition, the only one I have ever kept, and digging it out recently I was surprised to see how crammed and organised I had made my days. It is plain that I would allow no time to ruminate. I must be occupied.

I sent an account of my experiences to Jon back home. This is an edited extract, leaving out most of the art galleries and focusing on other things:

Paris lived up to my expectations and to the clichés. The city is a huge village across which you can stroll in an hour. The hotel staff seemed unfazed by the arrival of an entire department of bohemian English students bent on getting as quickly as possible to the nearest bar. Anthony and I were put into a small room with two skinny beds, foot-to-foot, and no toilet. There were no baths in the hotel either and the showers were often locked. Unpleasantly close to my pillow was a bidet. It was all very French.

In contrast to England the weather was hot and the skies cloudless. We were sleeping with the windows open and from the back of the building came the sound of scolding mothers, wailing children, and the endless moaning of beaten-up police vans clattering around the streets.

We studied a Paris map over a bowl of breakfast coffee with croissants, highlighting in pen the various places of artistic and historic interest that we wanted to visit. I stuck to my plan to do something in the morning, afternoon, and evening and therefore saw a good deal of the town and its museums and open spaces. We walked almost everywhere and quite quickly I found myself getting my bearings. The street name-signs are all in blue-green-and-white — house numbers in blue-and-white. They are very beautiful, and quite different from those anywhere in England. 'Do not be deceived by the "zebra crossings",' I wrote in my diary, 'Cars do not stop.'

Like every city, Paris has its own perfumes.

Everywhere there was the smell of Gauloises Turkish cigarettes, the vanilla of the two-foot-wide crêpes sold by endless pavement vendors, and a peculiar French scent seemingly worn by everybody, which clung even to the money in my pocket. It is a fragrant aroma but when I tried to point it out to people they denied being able to detect anything.

Anthony's French is limited to the basic, *'Un paquet de Rothmans s'il vous plait.'* Mine is better, but not much. Nonetheless I did all the talking and all the translating, and it was exhausting. After a time he was able to manage *'Merci'*, as well as the cigarette request, but he had no interest in learning more. I like French: the rules of the language seem easier to grasp than the irregularities of English. I bought *Le Monde*, which was too difficult for me, so to start a bit of French conversation I asked a shop assistant for some cheese. *'C'est un boulanger, Monsieur,'* she said in astonishment.

Saturday is market day and lying about in baskets or on slabs were mountains of fish, vegetables of all sorts, and every kind of meat and sausage. Skinned rabbits with crimson eye sockets hung from hooks, twisting in the breeze. We walked down some small streets crammed with Greek restaurants and stumbled on a fairground roundabout. Looking for the Panthéon we went to the Sorbonne by mistake. We had a cold beer in a café and then walked into the gardens and watched the men playing boules while we drank a bottle of wine. A plastic bottle of quite drinkable red can be had from the supermarket for the equivalent of about a pound. For some reason Anthony missed his footing at the Galerie nationale du Jeu de Paume and fell down the steps. I didn't see the spectacle because I was trying to buy some postcards in the shop.

We visited the wonderful Musée Rodin, an eighteenth-century mansion in a very salubrious part of town — lots of architects and doctors round that area I should think. We helped a man push his car down a hill. ''Aving a 'ard time wiz ze goddam' weather,' he observed in good idiomatic American. We went up the only hill in Paris to the Sacré-Cœur and I had a look over the city through a telescope. There was a fuss in the road, where a large piece of masonry had fallen off a building — firemen and everything.

We climbed a steep slope to a park. The sun bearing down on us made us thirsty so we 'uncorked' a bottle of wine. To soak up the wine we ate a phenomenal amount of bread and cheese. Still thirsty we opened another and became terribly inebriated. We managed to get back to the hotel, where I fell down the stairs into the lobby. These French stairs are very dangerous.

In the evening we found ourselves in the Rue St-Denis, where we had to hack our way through a jungle of prostitutes. They look very like their King's Cross equivalents, though somewhat older and with a sleeker sense of dress. The favoured outfit seems to be shiny boots, very short fur coat, and plenty of make-up. We made our way back to the hotel in good time as we had a train to catch in the morning: a group trip to Chartres.

I watched dawn gather over the lift shaft across the alleyway at the back of the hotel. There was trouble at breakfast: no crockery, or food, or indeed anything. Irritated and in a hurry, I asked for the necessities using any vocabulary that came to mind. The waitress complimented me on my French, but I didn't understand her.

We sprinted to the Métro, where we spent ten minutes hunting for Montparnasse on the map. Unlike London's superb Tube diagram, I found the Métro map a complete shambles, a snarled ball of knitting. Finally we found the stop and got to the Gare Montparnasse with just minutes to spare. We ran like the wind and leapt aboard the train. This was all very bad for my nerves.

In a stiff breeze outside Chartres Cathedral we all had to listen to a long talk by Cliff from the art history department. He has a habit of turning his head away during the last few words of a sentence, so that half the party caught things like '... ain façade of the cathedral or not', while others heard 'You simply must see the very moving — whooooo', as his words were blown away on the breeze. I knew that mathematics, especially geometry, had played a central role in the design of the church, and that with little more than a pair of compasses and a straight edge an entire cathedral had been conjured from the simplest elements: the square, circle, and triangle, resulting in the unified proportions that echo around the structure. From the positioning of the altar to the patterns in the magnificent rose windows, number holds sway above the flux.

It reminded me of the work I did as a boy, dividing and subdividing circles.

Cliff didn't mention the beauty of the geometry. He was more concerned with what the bishop was thinking when Charles the Bald gave him an old shirt. That man could make any subject boring.

Back in Paris for dinner Diana recommended a restaurant she knew and, rounding up half a dozen of us including strawberry blonde Alice and boozy Charley Lindsay, she took us off to the Rue du Faubourg Montmartre, a baguette's throw from the Folies Bergère.

We had to wait in a queue outside but before long a suave maître d'hôtel showed us through the revolving door and up a spiral staircase to a discreet little balcony with a couple of tables. We could look down from the gallery into the well of the restaurant proper. 'Belle époque' does not begin to describe the romance of this place. High ceilings, polished wood, huge built-in mirrors, veined marble dados, linen napkins, and a clientele of Parisians including professional men seated opposite younger women, who may be their wives.

This is good traditional food at a truly marvellous price. No cut glass: plain French tumblers. You decide what you want and a grumpy waiter dressed in black bow tie, waistcoat, and long white apron scribbles your order on a huge sheet of newsprint that lies on top of the red-and-white tablecloths.

Charley speaks not a word of French but within a minute he had the swarthy waiter laughing and smiling, talking in sign language about the bet he had on for some horse race. I wish I had this social knack but I don't.

After coffee I needed to water my horse. I found that the gents had those curious holes over which one is, presumably, meant to squat.

'How come those two footprints?' asked Rick.

'One for each foot,' said Charlie.

On the evening of the last day there was a knock on the door. To my immense surprise it was Alice, and Janice too, each holding a bottle of rosé. We invited them in and everyone got as comfortable as they could on the floor, on a bed, or on the edge of the bidet. We polished off the two bottles and finished the remaining beer and wine from our wardrobe 'cellar'. From time to time I caught Alice looking at me from the corner of her eye. I must have nodded off. When I awoke the room was dark so I crawled between the sheets and was gone to the world.

It was a terrible night. I woke repeatedly, tied up in the sheets and sweating like a horse. At about two o'clock I heard the sound of a person urinating in the washbasin.

Morning broke heavily. It looked as though someone had come in during the night and stirred the contents of the room with a giant spoon. The sheets were wine stained and there was a cigarette burn on the wall. My pillow was nowhere to be seen, my head was thumping, and I was gasping for a drink of water. As I got out of bed I trod on an empty tin of snails in garlic butter.

I threw on some clothes and padded off to the shared lavatory along the corridor. This toilet never flushed effectively. When you pressed the strange foreign mechanism it just boiled the contents into an unsavoury cassoulet.

When I got back to the room I discovered Janice clambering unsteadily out of Anthony's bed, sheepishly pulling on her bra. I wished her a dry-mouthed good morning and got a grimace in return. She pushed off back to her room.

Anthony emerged from the sheets looking damaged.

'Sleepless night?' I asked him. He said he felt as if his head was bigger than normal and that people were playing drums somewhere. I packed slowly, feeling wobbly.

My final diary entry read, 'Should be okay on the boat with enough fresh air and not too many head movements.'

Back home the crying man who wore kilts had moved out of the house, Tim Scattergood was still notching up women on his bedpost, and Reggae Man continued to play his deafening music. The antidote was my own handful of LPs. I particularly enjoyed the music of J. S. Bach, especially when played by a strange and brilliant pianist called Glenn Gould, who insisted on always performing on the same chair even after the seat fell out. I didn't know then that Gould's hatred of handshakes, his wearing heavy overcoats indoors, his health anxieties, his repeated nighttime egg meals, and his many other eccentricities were autistic signs, I just loved his idiosyncratic playing. Among other LPs in my collection were recordings of Gregorian chant, Spanish guitar music, and the lute works of John Dowland. But, as Sherlock Holmes says, 'To the man who loves art for its own sake, it is frequently in its least important and lowliest manifestations that the keenest pleasure is to be derived.' Thus I enjoyed military bands and sea shanties, and often played records of fairground organs, tin-whistles, and bagpipes. I sought out recordings of other unusual instruments, from the glass harmonica to the serpent, zither, and autoharp and would sit and listen to sound effects LPs as though they were music. I liked music hall songs, and had a collection of the signature tunes of radio and television programmes, going back decades, many of which I can still hum.

I liked character comedy and listened to Gerard Hoffnung reading out letters written in hilariously mangled English, which he claimed to have received from the proprietors of Tyrolean hotels: 'There is a French widow in every bedroom, affording delightful prospects ...' I listened to Joyce Grenfell as 'Shirley's girlfriend' discussing her boyfriend Norm, 'the one that drives the lorry with the big ears'. On television I saw Kevin Turvey, a character played by a young actor named Rik Mayall. He sat in a swivel chair and spoke in urgent non-sequiturs about cornflakes and the meaning of life. He had a Birmingham accent and mad staring eyes. Always it was silliness and the playful use of language that made me laugh.

Whenever I could, I liked to visit the typography department up at the main campus, where they sometimes held exhibitions of students' work: everything from book jackets to the design of individual letterforms and punctuation marks. The full stop at the end of this sentence is not just a dot; it was drawn by someone. I was particularly taken by what they were doing to improve the look and legibility of official forms. The proper design of forms demanded, like the cathedral at Chartres, a system of mathematical rules governing proportion: a set of cardinal precepts that insisted on nothing less than the pinnacle of clarity. Many people found these forms tedious, but I saw in their hidden design a deep abstract beauty. After a look round on my own I would return to the art department, my anxiety greatly reduced and my admiration for the skill and artistry of the typographers increased.

But still in my soul it was drizzly November and I traipsed around town trying to understand. I went on my own to hear Segovia playing at the venue where I had interviewed Barney Kessel. I wandered down Canal Passage, the road sign of which was frequently vandalised by the deletion of the letter C. Walking through the abbey ruins one night I heard a noise. In the gloom I could just make out the vague shape of a couple leaning against the remains of a flint wall, doing what people have always done in such places. I went into a pet shop, where I bought two zebra finches in a large cage: large for my room but too small for them to do more than flutter from one perch to the other. A cruel cage I now think. For quite some time they were to be my company, my friends.

One morning in the studio Big Lil poked her huge face round my partition.

'Tom,' she asked, 'how do you make brown?'

Was she serious?

'What sort of brown?' I asked, 'Raw sienna ...? Burnt umber ...? Cadbury's Flake?'

'You know ... brown.'

Having clear in my mind the memory of the typographers' deep understanding of their subject I was staggered that a painter at the end of the third year of a four-year fine-art degree course did not know how to mix a basic brown, the recipe for which infants stumble upon at school.

'Red, yellow, blue,' I said, giving her my best Pan Am smile.

I asked Tony the technician to erect partitions all the way round my area. I was now almost completely boxed in. Here I beavered away, producing the work for my degree exhibition, undisturbed and undistracted.

One day I found that someone had pinned an anonymous note beside my small painting, *Portrait of a Gibbon*, praising it extravagantly and offering to buy it. Was this intended to be amusing or nasty? 'That's Alice's handwriting,' said Anthony. But why would Alice, who seemed entirely indifferent to me, bother? There was nothing to lose so I responded with my own note, writing that as a member of the Expensivist school I doubted whether the picture was within the range of the prospective buyer. It was my first spoof letter. In the years to come there would be more, and better. I waited till the studio was clear and pinned the paper in Alice's space.

Later in the day there was a tap on my partition. It was Alice, wearing a clingy woolen jumper. 'Thank you for your reply,' she said. 'I'm not interested in buying your picture any more.' She burst into laughter. Her teeth, I noticed, were very neat. 'I hear there's a spare room in your house,' she said. Within two days she had moved in.

Alice would borrow teabags and she started to chat to me about painting and life. She laughed at my funny remarks without taking offence, or saying that I had a strange sense of humour, or was the rudest man she had ever met. One evening after a day in the studio she walked home with me. She spoke about her family and then, idly, about her boyfriend, who was, she mentioned quite casually, no longer on the scene.

Aha!

She came in for a chat. She was wearing a pair of tight trousers with vertical yellow and green stripes. Her strawberry blonde hair touched her shoulders. Instead of sitting in a chair she sat on the bed. I sat beside her, at a discreet distance.

I made some tea and we shared a couple of crumpets, then I showed her a magic trick. She wanted to see more so I did another and sat down beside her again. She took off her socks and wiggled her toes. I was very aware of her succulent perfume, which filled the crackling air. Neither of us spoke. Misjudging things badly, I lunged, smothering her and knocking over the bedside lamp. She became silent and still. I backed off.

'You can't just do this, you know,' she said sternly.

I subsided onto the floor, leaning deflated against the bed. Once again I had got the codes mixed up and put my foot in it. I was no good at seduction, no good at flirting and games. The business flummoxed me. Instead of logarithms at school how much more useful it would have been had we studied the rules of courtship. Alice got up and left, closing the door with a click.

I poured the tea dregs down the sink. Why was Tim Scattergood never flattened like this? I opened some sardines and ate them standing up, as I often did, straight out of the tin. Decades later I would read that the neurologist and 'honorary Asperger' Oliver Sacks used to eat sardine meals in the same way. I thoroughly washed the crumpet plates and threw the tin into the rubbish outside. Then I heated some lemongrass oil to perfume the atmosphere.

I picked up a book and read some extracts from the diary of John Dee telling of the strange behaviour of his nurse, who, on 29 September 1590, 'long tempted by a wycked spirit … most miserably did cut her owne throte'. It was plain from the story that this wycked spirit was what modern psychiatrists would call clinical depression.

There was a tap on the door. It was Alice. Her eyes were huge.

'You can stay tonight. If you want,' she said quietly, turning and padding down the stairs.

★

The next morning in the art department I was talking to Anthony as Alice came in. I winked and her cheeks flushed excitingly.

We bought bottles of wine and stayed in. We huddled under my umbrella in the hurtling rain. We ate our lunch in the park or spent sunny days on the river, watching kingfishers flashing across the surface. We dozed in the breezy grass under the willows. We went to the Bull and wandered home beside the riverbank casting long shadows in the golden sunlight. One day we swam among the reeds, Alice's mermaid body twisting like a silken rope.

At the house, Alice pointed out a cockerel strutting about the back garden under the trees. She said he was 'Gregory Peck'. He stayed a couple of days. I liked birds. Birds were wise, remote, but not unfriendly. Some would peck seed from your hand. Corvids used tools.

'Anthony told me you bought your zebra finches when you were sad,' said Alice. I smiled. As Jerome K. Jerome remarked, there is sometimes no language for our pain, only a moan. In *Three Men in a Boat* he tells a fairytale.

> Once upon a time, through a strange country, there rode some goodly knights, and their path lay by a deep wood, where tangled briars grew very thick and strong … One knight of those that rode, missing his comrades, wandered far away, and returned to them no more; and they, sorely grieving, rode on without him, mourning

229

him as one dead … One night, as they sat in cheerful ease around the logs that burned in the great hall, and drank a loving measure, there came the comrade they had lost, and greeted them … He told them how in the dark wood he had lost his way, and had wandered many days and nights, till, torn and bleeding, he had lain him down to die.

Then, when he was nigh unto death, lo! through the savage gloom there came to him a stately maiden, and took him by the hand and led him on through devious paths, unknown to any man, until upon the darkness of the wood there dawned a light such as the light of day was unto but as a little lamp unto the sun … And the name of the dark forest was Sorrow; but of the vision that the good knight saw therein we may not speak nor tell.

Alice, understanding, had led me from the depth of the forest out into the sun. I told her I wasn't sad any more. We decided that after our final exams we would move to London together.

★

In the last two months of the course we had to make final preparations for our degree exhibition. Charley, who had little to show for four years' 'study' got himself a vast roll of canvas and several washing up bowls, which he filled with paint. Nailing numerous sail-sized pieces up on the wall he brushed the paint over them with a long broom, never mind the drips. Once dry they were nicely stretched for him by Tony the technician.

I caught Charley off guard one afternoon beside his huge splodge-covered canvases. 'This is just a load of rubbish Charley, isn't it!' I said, in my usual unvarnished way. He smiled an intriguing smile. His final show made a big impact, but only really because the paintings were so enormous.

One of the visiting teachers in the art department was Adrian Heath, a great friend of Terry Frost, of the bowl of cherries fame. Being, like Frost, well heeled and well known, Heath was sycophantically admired by the teaching staff. One afternoon I was hanging my degree show: paintings of people and things with baleful atmospheres and titles like 'Mrs Febland Becomes Conscious of Her Own Mortality'. Austin Randall, who had always hated my stuff, was leading Adrian Heath through the studios to show him somebody else's work and was obliged to come through my space. Heath stopped in front of one of my paintings, one that Austin particularly loathed.

'That's a very good painting,' said Heath, looking it over for a couple of minutes. '*Very* good.' Austin caught my eye. I smiled a Cheshire cat smile. He was beside himself with fury.

The class of degree you were awarded hung on the whims of the teaching staff. A dissertation was part of the assessment process so I deliberately inserted three pages upside-down in various places, and stuck a couple of pages together with a dab of Cow Gum, a now defunct latex cement which you could roll into huge bouncing bogies. The dissertation came back with the pages still upside-down and stuck together. It had not been read. I didn't make a scene; my mind was already on London and getting away.

Boozy Charlie and Big Lil, who couldn't make brown, got very good degrees, as, quite properly, did Anthony. The tutors could hardly give me a final punishment beating or the vice chancellor would be down on them like a falling piano. So they damned me with faint praise, awarding me a middling degree. I decided not to go to the ceremony in the Great Hall to kiss the vice chancellor's ring, or whatever it was, and they posted the certificate to me. The envelope was less sumptuous than the one the vice chancellor had caused to be hand delivered all that time ago. I slipped out the certificate, gave it a look, folded it in quarters, and dropped it in the bin. In none of the jobs I was later to do did anybody ever ask to see it.

My old friend Jon, who was still at the Slade, asked if Alice and I would like to move with him into a large flat he had found in north London. I looked at my prospects. I had no money, no promise of any kind of job, and a degree that qualified me for nothing. But London flats were much cheaper then, and attitudes were different. Thousands of graduates were to be found bumming around the city before deciding what it was they wanted to do with their lives, while others squatted happily in a fog of joss stick smoke.

At school it had seemed that everybody was on my side. At university I had learned that many people were not. It was a sobering lesson, and one which knocked off a little of my naivety. I was eager to get away and I knew that in London, 'the Old Smoke', I would be among friends. Bill Bradshaw was already living in a wheelchair-adapted flat in Waterloo. Diana had bought a place in Stoke Newington and Anthony was going to move in as her tenant.

I cannot remember whether Alice and I worried about how we would pay the rent on an income of zero, but a dictum of the fourteenth-century Christian mystic Mother Julian of Norwich came to mind: 'All shall be well, and all shall be well, and all manner of thing shall be well.' I found this an uplifting maxim, and always have. Things would be okay. Something would turn up. London would be an adventure. I looked at Alice. She nodded purposefully. We told Jon yes.

Gazing across the pink roofs of the town, lightning flashes of memory lit up my mind: the dirt under Austin Randall's nails; Mr and Mrs Chambers dressed in their 'refinery'; Anthony falling down the steps of Paris; Alice's smile; and the vacant Fleeta Swit ambling across the quad, a pennant of toilet paper fluttering from her shoe.

I had long sensed that I was somehow different, but now, for the first time, I realised I could be happy. I squeezed Alice's hand.

'Whatever happens in future, if I seem … if I can't …'

'What?'

'You will forgive me, won't you?'

She laughed and threw her arms around me.

'Come on,' she said.

'Where to?'

'*London*, silly.'

We picked up our stuff and shut the door.

Chapter 5:
Road narrows

If a man does not keep pace with his companions,
perhaps it is because he hears a different drummer.
Let him step to the music which he hears,
however measured or far away.

HENRY DAVID THOREAU

For many years, flocks of artists, musicians, and students had been drawn to the 'urban village' where we had moved, warming to its cheap bedsits and convenient pubs. Though the first flickers of gentrification were becoming visible — a fancy café here, a skip on the pavement there — we felt at home in this bohemian corner, just five miles from the centre of London.

The flat was on the ground floor of a purpose-built post-war block at the top of a hill. It was a roomy place, easily big enough for Alice, Jon, and me. It was clean, well maintained, and regularly painted.

At the foot of our hill, God had pushed his thumb into the clay, making a dip in which the village had grown up. A banded clock tower crowned with a weathervane stood at the hub with roads radiating out like the legs of a spider. Going anywhere from this point meant climbing a hill.

I went for a walk past a disused Victorian–Gothic church which was to become a friend. I would give it a pat whenever I passed and say a few words, just as I had done with the lampposts of my youth. I found I could form reliable relationships with buildings. Being objects rather than people, they never confused me. This attitude is not uncommon for those on the autism spectrum. Wildly amusing autistic lecturer Ros Blackburn has even described the sexual affair she had with her ice skates.

I am reminded of a day, years ago, when I was on the beach with one of my nephews, a toddler who has some autistic traits. We were throwing pebbles into the water, and I explained how the receding waves tended to drag them out to sea. He looked anguished. 'I don't want to throw them any more,' he said. I wondered what was wrong and then the penny dropped. 'Oh, I forgot to tell you,' I said. 'When the waves come back in they bring the pebbles back onto the beach again.' He thought for a moment and resumed throwing. He saw the lonely helpless pebbles being dragged out to sea in the same way another child might see a person, or a pet rabbit.

I registered with an irrepressible doctor whose father had been murdered by the Nazis, and made an appointment with my new bank manager to discuss transferring my account and getting a chequebook. These then routine meetings now read like archaic rituals officiated by gentlemen in top hats.

One night we got back late to the flat. When I opened the door the floor seemed to part like a torn sheet. The carpet was a mass of cockroaches scurrying for their burrows under the sudden brilliance of the hall light.

We tried deadly powders and sticky insect traps, we complained to the management and made little headway. In the end, since the greasy insects never crawled across the dinner table or dropped onto our faces in the night, we learnt to live with them.

I got a job working with children in a play centre near Marble Arch. The money paid the rent and I was spending most of my time away from the hall of mirrors of adult life.

The area was a mixture of poor and rich families. There were youngsters from the Lisson Green estate as well as the sons and daughters of diplomats from the Mayfair embassies. Some children could name the countries of the world and speak French, Urdu, or Persian. Others could barely read. The tiny mother of one of the quieter girls worked at St Mary's hospital, nearby.

'What does your mummy do?' asked a nosey parent.

'She cuts up dead bodies,' replied the girl.

On a trip to the Kent countryside one boy saw his first cow.

A family of four Ugandan boys used to visit: David, Stephen, Silver, and Timothy. Silver was able to put his entire fist into his mouth, to the great delight of everybody who saw the performance. Their father Musa, a self-possessed, dignified man, looked after his sons on his own, having left his wife in Uganda the day he brought them to England.

One day, we were on an organised trip to the Imperial War Museum and, as I rounded a corner with the Ugandan boys, a display case housing a stack of First World War rifles came into view.

They froze, clapping their hands over their ears in terror. I had to lead them out into the fresh air.

Back at the play centre, their father asked if he could have a quiet word. I took him to a private room and we sat down. He told me about his country during the dying days of Idi Amin's dictatorship, where he had been arrested and imprisoned for I don't know what. He said he had been repeatedly beaten and made to parade daily with the other inmates while a uniformed solider came down the rows, whimsically picking out the men to be shot that morning.

One day, the soldier stopped in front of him. 'I know you,' he said. Musa looked straight ahead. The man pulled him out and marched him towards a building, where he shoved him into a dingy room and closed the door. This was it. The soldier spoke to him in an urgent whisper. 'You helped my brother,' he said. 'Go! Leave! Take your family.' He unlocked another door and pushed Musa out of the prison. 'Cover your face at the airport,' he hissed. 'They will see the bruises.'

Musa gathered his children and a hatful of money, wrapped a scarf around his disfigured face, and bought five tickets out of the country. He could not take his wife; she would join him later, they hoped. Shaking with fear, he made the long walk across the airport tarmac with his boys. He was not stopped. He climbed the steps and boarded the plane.

As Musa came to the end of his story a single tear ran slowly down his cheek. I was very affected but I did not understand how to express my mood. My face remained blank. I could never have touched his arm, much less embraced him. We returned to the playground so he could collect his boys, for whom museum guns were not neutral objects. They flung themselves around him.

Life in the flat ran smoothly. Jon was busy at college and Alice and I tended to do our own thing, especially at weekends. We would walk into London or go to the pub. Sometimes we visited Brighton for the day or took our sketchbooks into the park. After a few months we decided to look for a place of our own.

In those days, flat hunting was done with the aid of newspaper ads and a copy of the *A–Z* map book. Someone had also given us the name of Eugene at the Busy Bees Agency, which tracked down flats for people. I rang him from the work phone, which had a pale brown body and a darker brown handset. He found Alice and me the perfect place: a first floor flat on a busy crossroads, a mile north of Euston. An elevated section of the North London line passed close by the living room window. Trains chugged by all day over an ugly Victorian bridge while lorries thundered underneath, being supplanted at night by screaming police cars and singing drunks. For a person so sensitive to noise and overstimulation it seems curious that I could stand all this, but the urban bustle merged into a background rumble. I found it deeply romantic and slept soundly. It was the quiet nights and hooting owls of the countryside that drove me bananas.

The flat was above a knocking shop dressed up as a massage parlour. I would meet the girls shopping for cigarettes and sandwiches, and hear about their sore feet. We were flanked by a pie, mash, and eel shop and a small sausage factory, which, every Wednesday, took delivery of mountains of white pork belly dotted with nipples that would nevermore suckle a piglet.

One night, when I was about to push off to bed, the doorbell went. I trotted down in my dressing gown, and there, silhouetted against a streetlamp, stood the figure of a middle-aged man in a suit. He looked me over doubtfully.

'Do you do massages?'

'Next door,' I said.

'What, *sausages?*'

'Other side.'

In an upstairs flat lived two young men; the balding father of one used to present serious programmes on television. I passed him once on the landing as he went up to see his son, his crisp suit and tie clashing with the dust, shredded stair-carpet, and unopened bills that littered the floor.

We tried the pie and eel shop. The food consisted of a yellowish meat-filled pastry, served with dollops of watery potato engulfed in 'liquor', a hot sauce purportedly made with parsley and boiled eel juice, but actually just a flour gruel turned green by unholy quantities of food colouring. With your pie you could have a dish of hot, or jellied, eels. The jellied variety looked like something from an autopsy so I tried the hot ones. My disgust mechanism is finely attuned and the sensation of sucking the flaps and scraps off the snake skeleton made my skin creep. 'Why do you criticise everything?' asked Alice, not angrily but in search of understanding. I didn't know and couldn't say.

My zebra finches were getting on a bit, but they still hopped from perch to perch and squawked happily, or it might have been aggressively, whenever I put Gerald Finzi's *Dies Natalis* on the record player. Through Finzi's settings I discovered the haunting poetry of Thomas Hardy, whose novels I had always found so tedious. Finzi and Hardy remain golden threads uniting Then and Now in the ribbon of my life. Not long afterwards, both my birds died: first one, then the other. I felt the loss for a long time but kept the feeling a secret.

Alice got a job as an artists' model. When someone asked me whether I was happy with a lot of people looking at my nude girlfriend I said that what counted was whether *she* was happy with it. I knew that an artist in the studio becomes as emotionally detached as a surgeon performing a breast examination. Alice worked in the London art colleges and wherever else people needed a model. One day one of the ladies from a drawing class near Hampstead gave her a lift home. She told her that her husband Freddie had written a thriller called, *The Day of the Jackal*. Had she heard of it?

Somebody from Madame Tussaud's rang to ask Alice to model part of the torso of a young actress called Nastassja Kinski, who had not had time to sit for the sculpting of more than her head. They cast her hands and forearms using dental alginate. How strange to think that hundreds of thousands of people would soon be traipsing unknowingly past replica bits of my girlfriend. Somewhere today there are tucked away in forgotten holiday albums around the world a few faded snaps of Alice's young limbs. Would I recognise them?

I went to see Bill Bradshaw in his wheelchair-adapted flat in Waterloo. He was doing an office job which he was not enjoying and every spare moment was spent working on his linguistics PhD. 'My typist is making life difficult,' he complained. 'She says she can do it faster on one of those word processor things.' We went to the pub, where Bill drank a phenomenal amount of beer and smoked thirty cigarettes. Then we went for a phaal. He had always been quite good at eating.

I visited Jon at his new flat. He told me that Katy, the *belle* of my schooldays, had won a prize for the best English First in the University of London. I didn't doubt it. She was now at Oxford, being supervised by a divorced and remarried Catholic Marxist with money. It was not that Katy had an especially sparkling intellect, just a steely dedication to hard work, a canny awareness of the zeitgeist, and bulletproof ambition.

I thought I would like to work in radio but had no idea how anyone might go about doing that. In the end it was, as it so often is, a contact that put me on the path.

My aunt had just finished a short course in broadcasting techniques at an establishment near Harrow. She explained that they ran a highly regarded three-month residential course costing several thousand pounds. This was beyond me, but she said they were looking for someone with a bit of experience and technical nous, whose fees and room-and-board they would provide if that person would stay on to do a modicum of teaching and a fair bit of chair stacking during shorter courses throughout the year.

This sounded ideal, but there was just one thing. My aunt was a nun and the course was run by the Catholic Church. As a boy, I had been schooled by nuns, gone to church, learned the ropes. But this was all a long time ago. I sent them a letter anyhow and was invited along for an interview.

The journey into the outer suburbs on a musty slam-door train took me through Queen's Park, Wembley, and Harrow. I admired the Victorian terraces and red-brick suburban station buildings as we passed. When I wasn't gazing out of the window I was examining the seat moquette, a word coined in the thirties for the thick pile fabric used in upholstery. This one was hardwearing but unbeautiful.

I have an enthusiasm for public transport visual design systems, from typography to maps to cushions, and I often compare one with another. I once thought of having a suit made using the red and yellow moquette of the London Routemaster bus but decided it would be too prickly. Some of the best moquettes in the world are those used since the 1930s on London's underground trains, which were part of a sustained policy of integrated company design initiated by Frank Pick, the dynamic leader of what became London Underground. *The Oxford Dictionary of National Biography* describes Pick as 'very shy' and 'brilliant but lonely'. He was also highly focused. It was he, who in 1913 commissioned the calligrapher Edward Johnston to design the now world-famous Underground 'bullseye' roundel, along with a new typeface that would unify the look of all Tube trains, stations, maps, posters, and travel information. His idea was that attractive design, high functioning and well administered, can reflect an organisation's ethos and exert a profound effect on public impression. 'The test of the goodness of a thing,' said Pick, 'is its fitness for use. If it fails on this first test, no amount of ornamentation or finish will make it any better ...' He applied his 'bold simplicity' to everything from fabric design to the architecture of his new Tube stations, overseeing every feature down to the last fixture and fitting. The designer Noel Carrington thought his attention to detail made him the 'ideal inspector general'. Coherence, standards, and underlying systematic rules meant everything to him. I imagined Frank Pick on his cloud looking down at the seat covers of my train and cursing it.

The radio and television training centre was based in two huge 1920s houses in an affluent suburb a couple of miles from the end of the Bakerloo line. I was greeted at the door by a portly silver-haired man wearing a cravat and a signet ring. He said he was the dean. I said who I was. Exuding an aura of great suavity, he picked up the phone — a modern one, with buttons instead of a dial — and buzzed the person whose name I had been given.

'There's a sinister-looking young man here to see you,' he said, looking at me archly over his half-moon spectacles.

I was asked to wait, so I inspected the entrance hall. Ahead of me, a wide curled staircase led to two floors of accommodation, on my right was an office. Through a door to my left I could see a hotel-style sitting room with several armchairs. There were other doors but they were closed. From somewhere came the delicious smell of soup. After a minute a young woman with a beautiful smile appeared. She greeted me warmly and told me her name was Lea. This seemed a funny name for a woman. Lea was American. Perhaps this was why she seemed so effortlessly buoyant and upbeat. I liked her immediately. Of course I had no clue that this was my first meeting with my future wife. Who does? She told me she would give me a tour.

Hidden away inside the building was a large lecture room, a suite of offices, a chapel with access for cameras and microphones, and a full-size sound studio with a large control cubicle on the other side of a soundproof glass. My nerdy traits were immediately excited. Most astonishing was a huge, fully operational TV studio equipped with three cameras, lighting grid, cycloramas, and a control gallery housing a desk bristling with faders, buttons, and tiny lights.

I was interviewed by two of the staff before being taken to see the boss, Peter, a canon of Westminster Cathedral. He had something of the later Trevor Howard about him, his sideboard bristled with bottles, and his office clock had only one hand: 'one-ish, two-ish, three-ish', it said. After a bluff chat, Canon Peter saw me out and told me they would be in touch.

Back at the flat there had been a rustling under the floorboards and we noticed tooth marks in an aubergine. Mice! Hearing a noise in the kitchen, Alice opened the cupboard door. 'Argh! Tom,' she called, 'it's not mice, it's a huge rat.' Cockroaches was one thing, rats another. The massage parlour had been overrun. The environmental people fixed the problem but I spent hours with a bucket of bleach, cleaning every last surface.

On Sundays there was a huge market up the road. Crowds packed the stalls, bands played in the pubs, and canal boaters stopped for a chat at the lock. There was little I wanted to buy but it was nice to spend time with Alice. She was very good with other people and was my buffer against them. She was also by nature kind. One day near Baker Street she approached a tramp asleep beside his hat on a park bench. She lifted the hat and deposited a packet of cigarettes and a five-pound note.

Wandering about under a dark arch at the market one weekend she drew my attention to some colourfully braided lengths of what looked like rope. 'Aren't these unusual,' she said, lifting them up for me to examine. At once the ropes were whipped out of her hand. They were the dreadlocks of a man who had been bending forwards examining some bric-a-brac.

Despite her social skills and her altruism, Alice had always a fiery temper, and more than once I found myself in conversations with flying crockery. Like other Aspergers I shrink from conflict. When one evening I was hit on the head by a shoe I began to wonder how much of this I should be expected to put up with.

A letter arrived from the radio and television training centre telling me I had been successful in my application. I decided I would live at the centre during the week and come home to Alice at the weekend. I handed in my notice and left for the distant suburbs.

★

The three-month radio and television training course covered everything from the way a television studio worked to how to survive a tricky media interview. A BBC producer called Helen Fry talked to us about features. She had worked on *Plain Tales from the Raj*, the radio programme I had admired. I was going to discuss it with her during the coffee break but I was put off by the press of other people and overcome by anxiety.

We were given an introduction to drama by a very experienced producer, who took all of us through a short radio play. Some students were chosen to act, others took turns directing, and I, of course, volunteered to do the sound effects. This involved little more than putting down some cups and saucers and pouring out the 'tea' — actually cold water. It irked me that such effects were often too loud or in some other way exaggerated, as if the sound effects person was concerned lest his or her day's work go unappreciated. I carefully underplayed it.

'*Excellent* sound effects,' said the visiting producer. I had seldom been so flattered, for this was Piers Plowright, the man whose sound montage on death I had been so taken with. I wanted to tell him how much I loved his work and explain my conviction that a radio listener could detect the difference between hot and cold liquid being poured into a cup, but again I was unable to open a conversation or introduce myself.

The director of a new television drama called *EastEnders* showed us how to produce a multi-camera studio programme. Whoever was directing had to make endless real-time decisions: cueing the actors, and instructing the vision mixer, engineer, cameras, sound operators, and who knows how many other people while sitting in a darkened control gallery in front of a bank of monitors.

For some reason that nobody knows, the camera takes a particular liking to certain people and I found I was better in front of it than behind. I could talk to a lens more easily than I could a person, and I didn't have to order other people about. Presenting a show called *Book Review*, I gave an excellent impression of myself, looking relaxed and competent while they fed into my earpiece the developing chaos in the gallery, as student directors and vision mixers got in a shouting muddle, floor managers wandered into shot, and everything that could go wrong did. The adrenaline under the eye of the camera kept me agile and I found I was able to concentrate on my script, take the director's cues, watch the clock, and process the background hubbub, without too many problems.

People with Asperger's syndrome notice and remember distracting information that others ignore, and they can do this without it damaging their performance. This so-called, 'non-selective attention' was reported by UCL psychologists Anna Remington and John Swettenham, who asked a group of Aspergers to find the letters N and X in a ring of indifferent characters. Any letters that appeared outside the circle were irrelevant and should be ignored. The test was against the clock. They found that Aspergers processed more of the distracting information — the letters outside the circle — than did typical people, without this making them worse at the main job. In fact, they were better at it. Clearly there are times when distractibility is an advantage.

The most permanently useful training I had on the course was in how to be interviewed. As with other Aspergers I can find it hard to master my thoughts when asked a question, particularly one about myself. When I was being grilled I would often give strange terse answers, as I did in life, or would trail off into inarticulate irrelevancies. Watching my lacklustre performances being played back was a brutal awakening.

I learnt that although a media interview looks like a real conversation it is a mere imitation, with its own strange rules. Once I had understood this, I found the process easier, and with much hard work I learned how to pretend to be me, and to use the useful politicians' trick of *responding* to questions rather than answering them. This technique was exemplified by General de Gaulle who once waved a sheet of paper at some journalists, saying, 'Gentlemen, here are my answers, now what are your questions?' Of course, you could take it too far. This interview training helped me decades later when I was obliged to do endless interviews to plug books I had written. The rules of mock exchange were clear, and I enjoyed the performing.

When the course finished I stayed on in my bedroom 'over the shop'. I did a bit of hospital radio and I was offered some reporting work with the BBC. It was nice to get a cheque stamped with their monogram — my first broadcast earnings. The rest of the time I was helping out on the short courses that ran throughout the year. These were often for foreign students, from Scandinavia, India, Europe, and several African countries. On one course it began snowing and some Ghanaian priests who had never seen snow put on their overcoats and went onto the lawn, where they danced like children.

On another course a lot of senior English clergy, including a future Cardinal Archbishop of Westminster, arrived to have their interview skills polished up. One or two were on the ball. Others couldn't remember the question or keep their earpiece in. Another time the genial and rather vague director of a publishing house that produced English translations of papal documents arrived. Lea helped him make a short film and I talked to him about the right sort of typography for his captions. Later I saw him coming out of the ladies' toilet.

Lecturing more philosophically about the media was a Dominican priest named Gerard Meath. I introduced myself to him and told him he had taught my father at Laxton School. He remembered both my dad and my uncle Ralph. I walked with him to the car park, where he hiked up his habit, revealing a pair of pink legs and brown sandals. 'These medieval garments weren't designed for the modern world,' he announced, climbing into his car, which I remember as a Triumph Spitfire but probably wasn't. Then, staring absently into the distance, he mused: 'You know what, Tom, there's nothing so stupid as a nun.' With a sudden roar he was away, leaving me standing in a cloud of amusement and exhaust.

Oddballs, it seemed, were attracted to the Church. Running one of the courses was a 'mad professor' called Leonard Chase, who had been at the BBC in the early days, working on the radio thriller *Dick Barton – Special Agent* and the first episodes of the TV police drama *Z-Cars*. He had been the person who suggested Valerie Singleton as a suitable presenter for *Blue Peter* and had finally been made the corporation's head of training. He told me he had once produced a magic show for television, becoming so interested that he had taken up the hobby himself. He showed me a mysterious effect in which he pushed a borrowed pen through his jacket without leaving a hole. I was baffled until he revealed that the coat was woven from a tweed so loose that the fibres would part to allow a pen through, before closing up again. Leonard was a member of the Magic Circle and he invited me along as a guest. In time, and after a terrifying examination, I too became a member.

Canon Peter, the radio and television training centre's boss, was a whisky priest of the old school, whose phenomenal swearing was enough to curdle communion wine. He flew a 1935 glider, which he drove to airports in a long box on top of his Renault 4. He knew all the best hidden-away restaurants in London, though he was himself no chef. On the cook's day off he offered to make dinner for Lea and me. This turned out to be three catering meat pies blackened to a cinder in the deep fat fryer, served with frozen vegetable cubes boiled to a pulp. The meal was accompanied by several bottles of excellent wine, most of which disappeared inside the canon.

Lea and I began spending more time together. We went on a long walk and were followed by a Siamese cat. We lit a fire in one of the building's old grates, producing a lot of brown smoke and not much heat. Lea sifted the chaff and grain of my character, kept what was worth keeping, and with a breath of kindness, blew the rest away. Little by little our relationship changed. Something had happened. I decided that I was going to have to talk to Alice.

That weekend I went back to the flat. There was a steady drizzle, the pie shop and sausage factory were dark, and a blustery wind was holding a wet sheet of newspaper against the glass of the massage parlour: 'More pressure on Kinnock,' it said. I walked up the dusty stairs in darkness because the timer switch had failed. I let myself in and began the most horrible conversation of my life. 'You're being very good about this, you know,' said Alice. But I felt I had stifled a baby. There was blood on my hands for a long time.

★

The Canon invited Lea and me to a proper dinner. Round the table were several people including a couple of senior BBC types. I was out of my depth, but Lea charmed them even after she had sent a pickled onion flying into the lap of the Head of Religious Broadcasting. She mentioned that she had got herself a job offer as a production assistant with the BBC Drama department. The other senior BBC man leant forward, 'Oh, you won't be wanting to do that for very long. Come and see me when you've settled in and we'll sort you out with something more suitable.' I was shocked that this was the way it worked.

I think it was at around this time that, while having my eyes checked, I became properly interested in the weird typographic characters that are used on the test chart. Like everyone, I had been having this same eye test since childhood and I noticed, again, how strange the letterforms were. Looking into things, I discovered that abstract shapes had traditionally been used, but that in 1862 a Dutch ophthalmologist, Herman Snellen, had developed his own alphabet, using capital letters, or, at least, what are designed to look like capital letters. In fact, Snellen's shapes are not true letterforms at all and anything typeset in them would be next to illegible. Their purpose is not legibility but the testing of visual acuity while allowing the reader to identify easily each shape that he or she can see — a huge leap forward.

Just ten letter shapes are used in the standard chart: C, D, E, F, L, N, O, P, T, and Z. Their idiosyncratic geometry makes the thickness of each letter stroke equal to the width of the white spaces in between, and each serif the same. The height and width of the letters are five times this measure. Though the test has been developed over the years its properties remain the same today, more than a hundred and fifty years after its first use.

The Snellen letters have a systematic beauty, which I come back to often. But whenever I explain all this to opticians they seem bemused.

I was discussing the Snellen chart with Lea, but her mind was elsewhere. Her visa was about to run out and she had to return to the States. We went and stood outside in the drizzly rain. She did not believe it would be easy to get permission to come back to Britain to work. There were tears. I suggested we could get married. She nodded. There were no stars, no candle-lit dinner, no gemstones, just the gravel of the wet drive.

Lea packed her bags and I said I would go with her to the station. The writer and comedian Barry Cryer lived round the corner and for some reason, which I now forget, his wife dropped us off. I saw Lea onto the train and went back to her empty room. She had left a bottle of hair conditioner on a glass shelf. I picked it up and read the back. It was tremendously quiet without her.

With church attendance in England on the brink of its dramatic decline, the writing was on the wall for the training centre. I would be moving out of the place shortly anyway, my year being up. It had been arranged for me to spend a month as a spear-carrier with a local radio station off the M1. On my last day I found myself at the breakfast table with Canon Peter and the dean, who was demolishing a pile of toast and marmalade in engrossed silence. 'This is where you came in,' said the canon.

I collected my possessions, held in a single rucksack. As I left, Canon Peter was roping his glider to the car. 'The year comes full circle,' he said, giving me an unexpected hug that I did not know what to do with. I turned and looked up at the dark window of Lea's room. The sun caught the twinkle of ice on the casement.

★

I know exactly where I was standing at three thirty-nine in the afternoon on Tuesday 28 January 1986. I was beside the news desk of the local radio station, preparing to edit an interview I had done with a local cobbler. In those days you recorded onto magnetic tape and to make an edit you had to cut it with a razor blade either side of the bit you wished to remove, before uniting the two ends with sticky tape. It was a precise mechanical job that I enjoyed immensely.

The news team were nearby, wondering how to announce the officially unconfirmed collapse of a local firm. 'Say they're "folding",' said the editor. 'Use that word.' Next to me, a TV monitor was transmitting coverage of the latest space shuttle launch.

All at once something caught my attention. 'Er, I think there's some big news happening here,' I remarked. One or two of them looked up but nobody moved. Being a mere 'attachee' to the station I was of very low status.

The door burst open and a reporter dashed into the room. 'Have you seen it?!' he panted. They shot round to the monitor. The space shuttle *Challenger* had blown up during launch. The crew must surely be dead.

'Right,' said the editor, 'Drop "Potholes". This is it for the four o'clock. Chris, find a local spokesman. Ronnie, get on to London and see what they've got.'

During my month with the station I did a bit of everything: recording trails, interviewing local celebrities, sitting in on tedious meetings. Princess Diana visited the town and my job was to sprint from reporter to studio and back again with reels of tape. I said things like 'Steve says the second vox pop is best' and got replies like 'Tell him to give us a three-two-one countdown on these for God's sake. We're pulling our bloody hair out.'

Some of the programme producers, including news producers, struck me as remarkably ill informed. They knew the ranks of the police force, the currencies of the world, and what you weren't allowed to say about court cases, but I had to tell various people at various times, a) who John Ogdon was, b) what ICI stood for, and, c) who composed *Peter and the Wolf*. Though many presenters were admirably quick on their feet I was disheartened by the contrast between their amiable joviality in front of the microphone and their brusque, humourless pushiness in the office. This two-facedness struck me as both glib and underhand.

I sent a thin blue airmail letter to Lea in America. 'It's working with people I'm no good at,' I said. 'The horror of meeting people is something I will never escape. I find it hard even to talk to them here. Perhaps I'm just bonkers.' I had been aware for many years that something funny was going on with me but this was the first time I had written it down.

I left the place without fanfare, deciding that a radio station which was little more than a jukebox with traffic reports was not the sort of radio I was interested in.

Since the cupboard was bare, my parents had dubiously agreed that I might stay with them for a short time. I scanned *The Guardian* every Monday looking for media jobs, but in the meantime I needed cash. I went for an interview at a family-run department store in a nearby spa town.

'We are the Harrods of the South East,' said the lady interviewing me.

'Surely Harrods is the Harrods of the South East,' I thought, but didn't say.

They put me in the gentlemen's outfitting department. I felt as if I had fallen into Grace Brothers, the fading department store of the BBC's *Are You Being Served?* I was given training in how to use a tape measure and also in something called, 'Being Positive', which amounted to pretending to be every shopper's friend. I didn't do very well at this. If I thought a garment didn't fit, looked ghastly, or was badly made I told the customer so, but it was explained to me that this was 'poor salesmanship'.

Despite their offensive propensity to lie through a smile, I found my colleagues to be more rounded, mature, and serious than my university cohort. They tried to show me how the world worked and this was good for me.

One quiet morning during the first week, my supervisor asked me to try on a jacket that a suit rep had given him. It was pale blue and the lapels were about a foot wide. It looked very unusual in the changing room mirror and I was sceptical.

'Is this right?' I asked through the curtain.

'Try the trousers,' he said, handing them through.

The trousers were of the same colour but would have made a sailor's bell-bottoms appear narrow. They were too long and the waist was loose. Looking at my absurd reflection the first inkling came upon me that I was being set up.

'Come out and let me look at you,' said my supervisor.

Clutching the waist of the trousers I waddled out from behind the curtain to find the whole team standing in a semicircle. A loud roar went up.

'I was *led*,' I said, 'Led, like a lamb to the slaughter.' It had been an initiation ceremony, and I had survived it.

The public areas of the shop were deeply carpeted but the staff stairs were cold and hard. Coming down them one day I passed the open door of the MD's office.

'What's a "mausoleum" and how do you spell it?' came a voice.

I stopped and put my head round the door. 'It's a big building with tombs in it,' I said. 'M-A-U-S-O-L-E-U-M.' To my astonishment the boss blew his top, sending me packing and screaming at me from the head of the stairs. What was the matter? He wanted information; I had that information; and I had given it to him, at no cost.

But there was a cost. I didn't understand it then, but I had made a social error of the grossest kind, severely undermining a person whose sense of self resided, perhaps exclusively, in his position as alpha male. To have a subordinate encroach on his territory and display evidence of superiority in front of another subordinate was excruciatingly damaging to his self-esteem. The omega male had urinated in the alpha male's lair. I try to be more careful now, but still put my foot in it from time to time. If you have Asperger's you tend not to pick up on these things as others do.

I sent a daily postcard to Lea, keeping her up to date with my thrilling adventures. 'They put me in charge of trousers,' I wrote. 'Hooray! This is so stimulating that I wouldn't be surprised if I woke up.' I knew that I wanted to spend my life with Lea and I was saving every ha'penny to travel to the States to get married. But marriage seemed a ridiculous business, and to me weddings were superstitious rituals unsuitable for a decent person to get himself mixed up in. I had made a private agreement with Lea. That was the important thing, not a public display.

Nonetheless, there were rational reasons to go ahead, the chief one being that I would mortally offend Lea's family if I did not. On the other hand, I could not invite members of my family or any friend. I could not even talk about it. I had no understanding of how hurtful this course of action was to be to my parents, Jon, and my brother and sisters, nor how puzzling it would be to my wife and my in-laws. It was possibly the most damagingly autistic thing I have ever done. I did not understand my motives and it would take decades for the light to dawn.

By early summer I had a plane ticket, but to be married I needed my birth certificate. I asked my parents where it was.

'Why do you need it?' they asked.

'Because I might get married,' I said, using the conditional tense to buffer the announcement. Naturally they were nonplussed, but all I could think about was my own discomfiture. What a truly hateful business this wedding nonsense was. How and why did people put up with it?

★

Girt by the vast expanse of flat grasslands of the Great Plains, the oblong state of North Dakota stands in the geographic centre of North America. If you hammered a giant nail into the cowboy-flavoured town of Rugby ND you could rotate the whole continent around it. The wide Missouri flows through the Dakotas like a liquid mountain, sparkling under the broiling sun or groaning beneath a foot-thick lid of winter ice. This is the country's oven, and its ice box. To the dark-red west the burning coal furrows of the northern Badlands let tufts of smoke into the huge skies. Before their destruction the Mandan, Lakota, and Hidasta peoples lived here. Their name for the area meant 'place of the tall willows'.

The plane was making its descent into the airport of the city — now improbably named Bismarck — the state's capital and Lea's longtime home. As we banked to port I spotted the capitol building below me, projecting from the surrounding flatness like the arm of a drowning man. After so many months I was about to see Lea again.

Coming out of the cool aircraft into the stifling humidity of the summer air I saw her waiting for me. She was smiling excitedly; her hair bleached by the sun. We were very glad to see each other.

She drove me home and I was inspected by family and friends. I tried to seem normal.

'He doesn't like to be hugged,' said Lea, '*because he's English.*'

I hit it off with Lea's mother, an energetic surgical nurse, and, more gradually, with her father, a generous host. He had worked as a midshipman on the Great Lakes freighter, SS *Edmund Fitzgerald*, which finally took her crew to the bottom of Lake Superior in a monster storm. He had been a union firebrand but wanted to talk about Chaucer. The opening of *The Canterbury Tales* had been drummed into me at school, so I was able to impress him by reciting it from memory over dinner.

Beyond the family, my accent was a cause of great interest and amusement. At the Ground Round restaurant on Third Street I tried to ask about their beer. I used every pronunciation known to phonetics but the waitress looked blank. I was obliged to write it down on a napkin. 'Oh, *beer*,' she said.

'Even when you swear it sounds so polite,' someone told me.

The visitors bureau described Bismarck as 'a hub of culture, history, and shopping'. Everything was somewhere else and you got there in a car. Directions were given by green highway signs crowded with ill-positioned blue shields containing ill-spaced yellow numerals. Next to these, on the same sign, were white Native American-head silhouettes, with black numerals on them indicating who knew what. So ill drawn were they that at even a short distance they looked more like squashed albino hedgehogs.

Lea took me to a cattle auction, with real cowboys chewing real jerky and buying real cows. We went bowling. The noises, and smells, and lighting were horrible, and I was obliged to wear special shoes that made me cringe.

Few locals ventured beyond the state, but everyone was on top of the world. Strangers greeted me warmly, and unlike his surly British counterpart the Pepsi deliveryman whistled with pride. You were not old, you were 'senior', and if you were wrinkled there was something you could do to defeat it. Life, and even, it sometimes seemed, death, could be tamed. My waitresses for today offered me expansive breakfasts of bacon, waffles, and syrup. 'Oh, hey, are you English?' or Irish, or Australian, they would gurgle. 'How cool.' Shortly before the wedding I was taken to be measured for a monkey suit. Could it be altered by next week? No problem. The constant sunny-side-upness was a refreshing change from the Northern-European stoicism I was used to, but it got a bit much. Checkout girls kept telling me to have a nice day, even when I had other plans.

We visited a pig farm where they dressed us in white scenes-of-crime outfits. We looked as if we were going to be handling plutonium. A thousand animals were squashed together in an unlit concrete hangar. Bowling balls had been provided to distract them from killing each other out of boredom and fury. There was no happiness in these nitrogenous sheds and we left. The smell of pig clung to our clothes and car for days.

Near the confluence of the Heart and Missouri rivers we saw the rebuilt house that General Custer had lived in until his unfortunate appointment at Little Big Horn. All around was the familiar prairie landscape I had heard about in the stories of Laura Ingalls Wilder, which my mother had read me when I was a boy. We visited the On-a-Slant Native American village, where the Native Americans were no more. Native American matters were handled, I learnt, by a government agency called the Bureau of Indian Affairs, or BIA, which stood, the Native Americans said, for, 'Bossing Indians Around'.

We were asked to speak to a class of English undergraduates at the university. They wanted to know about exchange rates, which jobs paid most in Britain, and my advice for getting on. 'Cultivate the art of doubt,' I said. 'Read a book. Think for yourself.' They looked blank.

We went to hear wedding organists demonstrating their skills. I was dumbfounded by their commingled incompetence and chutz-pah. A fat young woman stumbled through simplified wedding marches on a Wurlitzer in her dining room.

'Do you know any Handel?' I asked in desperation.

'Oh, are you an organist too?' she squeaked.

'No,' I replied, 'but I have heard of Handel.'

After slaughtering a stripped-down arrangement of *The Arrival of the Queen of Sheba* she turned to face us with a huge smile, mistaking my rictus of disbelief for approval. So bad was she that she thought she was good. I later learnt that this cognitive peculiarity has a name: the 'Dunning–Kruger effect'. It's a good one to remember. It seemed to be more pronounced here than at home.

I was staggered by the stuff that came out of the television. It was a freak show of wobbly soap operas and shouty commercials for one-cal root beer, spectacular storewide savings, and control-top pantyhose. 'Like sands through the hourglass so are the days of our lives …'

Clicking through the million channels I found the commercial-free C-SPAN (the Cable-Satellite Public Affairs Network), which was transmitting live pictures from the space shuttle that showed the astronauts doing science experiments. It was bliss to sit there for half an hour and watch two white-clad people drifting about holding weightless petri dishes and bits of foil. Almost nothing happened and it was mostly silent. Every few minutes the camera would cut back to Mission Control, where two or three people sat, scratching their noses. From time to time a quiet voice would ask a question or make a cryptic announcement. Like poetry it slooooowed you down.

I hadn't given Lea an engagement ring. It seemed irrational to waste money on a superstitious gewgaw. Why not give a woman something of value instead: a nice big potato, say, or some pens? Lea's father no longer wore his wedding ring so Lea decided to have it resized for herself. I am not a jewellery wearer or remembrance poppy flaunter but they told me the ceremony was to be a 'two-ring' affair, meaning that I also needed one. I went to a discount store resembling a low-grade Woolworths and approached the young man behind the counter.

'I want the cheapest wedding ring you've got.'

He drew my attention to a revolving mock-velvet display. 'This is a medium weight court ring, Sir,' he said, pointing with his little finger. 'Is that the sort of thing?' An aerosol of synthetic cinnamon blew across us.

'How much?' I said.

'A hundred and seventy five dollars.'

'How much is that one?' I asked, indicating a tin-coloured also-ran at the very bottom. I didn't have time to mess around.

'That one, Sir,' he said, making the face you might make when clearing rotting fish from a gully, 'is thirteen dollars and twenty cents.' I bought it, declining the fancy box. After the wedding it turned my finger black so I threw it away.

If I were to do all this again I think I would be more aware of other people's feelings about things like rings. For me and my autistic mind they had no symbolic meaning, purpose, or value. For many people, perhaps most, they do.

The night before the ceremony, the tuxedo arrived, swaddled in tissue paper. I tried it on. The trousers and sleeves had been painstakingly adjusted but everything was two inches too short, revealing my socks and half a yard of shirtsleeve. There was no time to change it.

Lea's father was pacing up and down, complaining that he was having a heart attack.

'Take one of your indigestion tablets,' said his wife, who, after a lifetime of nursing knew the difference between pre-nuptial anxiety and acute myocardial infarction. But his symptoms worsened and he was taken to the emergency room.

'What's going on?' he asked, clutching his chest.

'You're having a heart attack,' they said, and put him in intensive care.

On the morning of the wedding, I showered and decided to dry my long hair in the hot sunshine. This had the curious effect of making me look like the secret love child of Albert Einstein and Phil Spector. My brother-in-law, who was to be my best man, tried to damp it down but it was hopeless. He'd get it flat in one place and it would spring up somewhere else.

The venue for the service was a split-level 1970s fibreboard church, brutally carpeted throughout. We had rehearsed the evening before and the amiable young priest who was to be the celebrant took it well when I insisted on going through everything I would be called upon to say, so as to expunge anything I believed to be false.

On the day, there seemed to be special rules which nobody had explained to me. Moments before the ceremony I was admonished for eating a sandwich. Looking around the crowd as I stood on the carpeted platform, I realised that apart from Lea and her immediate family I knew not a soul.

We went to a local hotel for the reception. Lea's family's friends and relations came to shake my hand: university people, mechanics, elementary-school teachers. They wanted to chat. The whole thing was the typical Asperger's nightmare. Luckily there was alcohol to take the edge off. A local photographer took photographs of us holding bits of cake: me in the runt's suit, my long hair shivering in the air conditioning. But she did something wrong and the pictures came out so orange that we threw them away.

We drove some wedding cake to my father-in-law in the ER. He was plugged into bleeping machines and looked green. We stood briefly in the incongruous setting, Lea in her white wedding dress, me in my short-sleeved tux.

We had decided to travel to South Dakota for our honeymoon to take a look at Mount Rushmore, which Hitchcock used so brilliantly for the climax of *North by Northwest*. It was a long drive across the prairie, with the accelerator set on 'cruise'. There was sun, wind, and mile after mile of flat openness. We passed occasional small towns that seemed unchanged since the days of the Wild West but for the paraphernalia of the internal combustion engine. We were to stop overnight en route but because of a baseball match most of the hotels were booked up. At the last minute Lea had found us a motel and reserved a room.

It was dusk when we arrived. The owl that had been flying alongside us flew off as we pulled in. We could see this was not the ideal honeymoon place. Its dust, neglect, and yellowing net curtains made Bates Motel seem like the Ritz. We looked on the bright side and pushed on south next morning.

Seeing Mount Rushmore after dark was said to be dramatic, and hopes were high. A man gave us a fascinating talk about the monument's construction and announced that the lights would now be switched on to reveal the presidents in their glory. There was a deep clunk and we found ourselves staring up at a vast curtain of mist.

'You'll have to come back tomorrow,' said the guide.

Back in North Dakota someone asked if we would like to tour

the State Penitentiary. Not many honeymoons feature a prison visit so we said yes. We were shown around a newly built part of the jail. There were cells off a gallery from which you could look down into an open area. We were introduced to a polite inmate in a smart uniform, who proudly showed us his room. He was particularly pleased with the view from his arrow-slit window, out onto the parking lot.

'What's he in for?' I asked our guide afterwards.

'Raped an eight-year-old girl,' she said, looking for something in her handbag.

She took us through a locked door into a room where convicts were spinning pots and painting sunsets. Some were huge unsmiling Native Americans who were not in prison for parking violations. A few had murdered people. I felt uneasy. I was a skinny little thing accompanied by two women. The inmates spotted my strange demeanour at once, and had they decided to get nasty I don't think I would have lasted long.

On our way out of the building we passed a dim passage with a parade of squat old cells. Pacing like animals behind the flaking paint of their iron bars were the gloomy figures of caged men. It was nice to get out in the sunshine again.

Not much later we heard that the priest who had married us had been admitted to a mental hospital.

★

We returned to England with little money, nowhere to live, and no jobs. Lea's application for a work permit had been denied while we were in the States so she couldn't accept the BBC post. My patient parents put us up while I checked in with Eugene at the Busy Bees

Agency. One day a strange voice answered. Surprised, I said: 'Is that you, Gene? Um — is that you-you Gene? Er — is that Eugene?'

We liked North London so Eugene sent us to the purlieus, some less lovely than others. We turned up at a house near the Holloway Road, where the door was opened by a giant in a none-too-clean vest. 'You're early,' he grunted through broken teeth.

We were shown into the dark hallway. Off this uninspiring passage sprouted a kitchen with a filthy stove and a frosted plastic window onto somewhere else. The lino-floored sitting room contained a massive fridge covered in brown stains, and a vinyl sofa with foam rubber erupting from a long knife slit. The nearby lavatory was so narrow you would have had to back into it if you wished to take a seat. Everything smelt of fried onions. We were polite but didn't stay for tea.

We saw an attic flat in a half-timbered house in an Edwardian suburb near Alexandra Palace. It had a charming little kitchen and a decent size sitting-cum-dining room. If you stood on tiptoe you could peer from the skylight into the wood opposite. 'This is good,' I whispered. Lea seemed doubtful. She was used to American walk-in closets, en suite bathrooms, a carport, and a gym. In the end we took it and came to love it.

Now married to an Englishman, Lea was offered another job by the BBC. I continued to check the paper.

Like everyone else, almost all Aspergers want to work, but many of these frequently talented people end up with no kind of permanent paid employment. I knew that I struggled in interviews: misunderstanding the situation and making people feel awkward by my strange eye contact and Pan Am smile. I got the feeling when I was turned down for things, as I repeatedly was, that something had gone awry during the interview — as if I had used the wrong knife and fork during a royal banquet. I would sense the ice forming on their faces.

Employers tend to hire people who are like them, but Aspergers are not like anyone else: they are like themselves, and when the employer asks the question, 'Will this person fit in?' the answer is often a reverberant, 'No!' Though there are niches where autistic people can make a powerful contribution to organisations using strengths other than social facility, it's getting the job that is often the hard bit.

The UK's National Autistic Society has found that employers think autistics need solitary technical jobs requiring attention to detail. A good number do want jobs of this kind, but others do not. For example, as many autistics want to work in the arts as in IT, and this was true of me, though I did not know exactly what I wanted to do. Surely there must be a field for my particular powers, if only I could find it.

Plenty of people with autistic traits show strengths early on in the spheres they later go into professionally, and it is frequently the oddballs — those who had a miserable time of it at school — who end up with the most interesting jobs. Anthony Hopkins showed early promise as an actor, and the author E. B. White, who was troubled by noises and smells, and so fearful of public occasions that he was unable to attend his own wife's funeral, had always been interested in writing. He adored nature, and this, along with his love of children resulted in his classic *Charlotte's Web*. 'All writing,' said White, 'is both a mask and an unveiling.' He was fascinated by the systematic rules of language and, in typical pedantic style, co-authored *The Elements of Style*, a classic guide to English usage.

I too have always deeply enjoyed the pernickety details of style, and find etymology rewarding. A few years ago I discovered the

Online Etymology Dictionary, etymonline.com, the compiler of which is Douglas Harper, who has an enthusiasm for the history of Cleveland street railway cars. Learning this I felt the secret handshake of the Asperger and was unsurprised to find the following in his brief online autobiography: 'I was thought to be in need of remedial education for dyslexia; had the diagnosis of Asperger syndrome been known then, I have been told I might have been given that.'

★

Money was tight. We were eating a lot of cheap mince, and liver. I applied for a broadcasting job but botched the interview.

'Your application form is beautifully typed,' they said.

'My wife did that,' I replied.

I needed income. One evening in a pub the landlord heard me say I had done bar work.

'I can give you a job, if you like,' he said.

'When?'

'Now.'

On Saturday nights the place was packed and a band containing the *Punch* cartoonist Wally Fawkes pulled them in. I didn't get on with the other staff but the evenings went in a flash and I was reminded of my time at the hotel on the river.

Later, I managed a high-street toyshop in Islington. A collection of elasticated animal noses was delivered: pig, horse, cow. I arranged them in a basket and wrote a notice: 'Animal noses. Pick your own.' The actor Bob Hoskins came in and spent a fortune but was shirty when I wanted to verify his credit card. I sold the protean Michael Ignatieff a wind-up steam train. 'I thought you'd like that,' I said. In the middle of summer, I put out a big Santa Claus holding a sign: 'Only 173 shopping days to Christmas.' The job had its moments, but I was at a loss. The owner resented my querying her instructions and my assistant complained that I was insufficiently bossy.

I took a job at a lithographic printer's run by a man who combed his hair across from the back. When he went to the post it was blown into a vertical ginger flame. His ink-covered assistant ate a lot of cold sausage and taught me to fan paper, a skill with which I can still impress people. They put me behind the counter, dealing ineptly with customers who wanted things photocopied.

A mild little man asked me to copy some Polaroid pictures he had taken of himself wearing ladies underwear, and a famous actress wanted the whole of *Othello* reproduced. 'Cheaper if you do it yourself,' I said. There was an old soldier who frequented the place dressed in a smashed-up hat, disintegrating tie, and a threadbare shirt that poked out of the fly of his baggy trousers. His chin was a patchwork of smooth bits and rough bits and his broken glasses looked pre-war. But he was well scrubbed, smelling strongly of coal tar soap, and spoke in clipped officer-style tones.

'I must have this document copied,' he said. 'It's my letter to the Queen.' I looked down at the scrawl-covered ream of dog-eared sheets so thumbed and soft they barely hung together.

I didn't know what had gone wrong for this man, but he must once have been a normal little boy sitting down to tea with his mum or running about laughing with his playmates. Not knowing quite how to handle the situation I hesitated, but a colleague, one of the world's natural psychologists, stepped forward.

'We can do this for you, Sir,' he said, 'but you will have to leave it with us.' The man put both hands down on top of the papers and, like a cat with a kitten, drew them in protectively. He decided he would do it himself and was in the shop for hours.

One day a man in a black suit came in. He showed me part of a newspaper containing a two-column story. 'What do you think is wrong with this?' he asked in an insistent monotone. I looked it over and read it through. I didn't know what he was getting at. 'Look,' he said earnestly, not meeting my eye, 'the margin between the columns has a vertical rule in it. That's all wrong.' I must have looked puzzled. 'It's the space between the columns that is the separator, not the rule. The rule does not help: it confuses.' I made him five copies and he left.

On the way home I realised he had been making a point so dazzlingly obvious that it was impossible to understand without deep thought. His five minutes with me made such an impression that in all the work I did in later years I would object whenever a designer or typesetter tried to use a rule instead of space to separate columns of text. He was an odd, monomaniacal character, that man: a chap after my own heart. It is only lately that I have realised that he was showing definite traits of Asperger's syndrome.

On Saturday mornings Lea and I would potter about the flat, drinking tea. Standing on tiptoe and looking across to the wood I used to listen to a radio programme called *Loose Ends*, in which a fey academic named Professor Donald Trefusis sometimes presented, 'wireless essays' on serious subjects. This was, in fact, character comedy of the highest quality. I admired the way the writer–performer, whoever he was, attacked full-frontally the things and people that annoyed him. The anger-turned-to-laughter reminded me of the letters of Edna Welthorpe (Mrs). I could do that, I thought. I would be good on *Loose Ends*. Not that anyone was going to invite me. It was only years later that I discovered the name of this young performer. He was Stephen Fry.

We took weekend strolls around the suburb and I noted lampposts, bridges, and road signs. The signs were generally of the Kinneir and Calvert sort, but tucked away here and there one could find examples in the old style, which had evaded replacement. In one of these, the white arrowheads pointed to 'Highgate; Holloway; Finchley'. Something about the character of this twenty-year-old notice told of a time of bomb sites, trams, and tweeds. Against the classic faded blue background, the letterspacing of the bold black capitals on white oblongs was good, and the typeface admirably clear, but as a unified thing it just wasn't as effective as the new signs. Nonetheless, despite my love for the new, the muddle-through British charm of the quieter age shone out from the face of the old.

Lea had been at the BBC for a while, working on various dramas. She was good at the job, but the pay was feeble. One day the man I had seen coming out of the ladies' toilet at the radio and television training centre got in touch and offered her a job. He was the publisher of the Pope's encyclicals in England and wanted to expand into making and selling videos. The money was a good deal more than the BBC and there was a pension, so she said yes. After a while he needed a new editorial assistant and he offered me the role.

'I've never worked in publishing,' I told him.

'I'll teach you. I think you'd be excellent,' he said. 'And I'll pay you more than you're earning.'

I couldn't believe my luck. The work sounded fascinating and Lea would be in an office upstairs, so we could unwind on the Tube home. The new boss was a change from the printer with the vertical hair. He was a polished Brasenose graduate who read Latin, and seemed clear-headed, sane, and sensible. Little did I know.

I left the printer's and started at the publisher's, which owned a tall white building in a Pimlico square, minutes from Victoria station and close to the road where my mother had lived after her father's death.

'You will share an office with me,' said the boss. 'Here's a key to the garden.'

He was as good as his word, teaching me about book production and editorial matters. I was introduced to *Hart's Rules for Compositors and Readers* and learnt about 'Oxford style'. I found I was a natural proofreader who could spot a wrong-font hyphen at a thousand yards. I fell in love with the so-called 'Oxford comma', the much-argued-over, 'extra' comma before the last item in a list. I found some delicious examples of what could happen if you failed, or refused, to put one in: 'This book is dedicated to my parents, Gertrude Stein and God' and 'Alan Whicker's tour included meetings with Mother Teresa, an 800-year-old demigod and a collector of dildos.'

These were the fag-end days of hot-metal printing, a world populated by old men who could zero in on a *p* instead of a *q* in a tray of upside-down back-to-front type. From them I learnt about the craft of compositing and printing. My childhood days poring over sheets of rubdown letters came back to me. There was an inky magic to the business, which was shortly to be swept away by computers.

I sometimes ate my lunch in the beautiful garden in the middle of the square. The gardener, who wrote books on the subject, had a fondness for catapulting cables high into the plane trees, up which, over the years, he trained a forest of climbers.

I was guided around the publisher's stock room by two crones who had worked in the office since the war. Their life's meaning was to hate each other. As they bickered I looked through the backlist: apologetics, the lives of the saints, the *Catechism*, Church history. One day I recognised the cover of one of the pamphlets. It was a biography of Padre Pio, a priest who claimed to have had on his hands the bleeding wounds of Christ. It was the very booklet Bob Strange had shown me years ago in the art department refectory.

The company was full of unusual characters. Doing some sort of office management job was a woman who insisted on being called Bernard. Her face, a colleague told me, would change from green to blue whenever he walked into her office, as she clicked off the prototype poker website she was furtively using. In an attic room dwelt a tiny lady of about a hundred, who made tea for the boss in an iron kettle that weighed a ton because its interior was encrusted with two inches of pre-war limescale.

The quickest way from the editorial office to the stock room was down a very dark staircase that backed onto a yard. The rear of other houses at right angles to this one looked over the same space. As I ran down one day I glanced through the tall window that lit the stairs. Across the way was a brightly illuminated room and walking about inside it a young woman, completely naked. There was a delight in seeing this graceful figure unselfconsciously moving about in her space, unaware that she was being observed, but at the same time I felt a pang of protectiveness. It was an odd business.

One spring day, the big brown office telephone rang. It was a friend telling me of the death of the comedy actor Kenneth Williams. I remembered watching him during recordings of *Just a Minute* and thinking there was something very weird about the man. He was a terrific raconteur but he grimaced and scowled, and refused to drink the BBC water, calling it, 'foetid'. He was noticeably remote, using very restricted eye contact, and accepting handshakes and the odd hug without enthusiasm. A cold fish. His editor Russell Davies called him 'a strange and dislocated person-ality', while his revealing diary, which he said eased his loneliness, recorded in perfectionist detail his isolation and constant health anxieties: notably his bowel problems.

In his areas of special interest, including history, typography, etymology, and the rules of English usage, Williams was erudite. He loved maps and as a youth had been an apprentice at Stanfords, the London map company, before joining the Royal Engineers as a map draughtsman. He was an enthusiastic reader of non-fiction and poetry, but a stranger to bookshops and libraries. He read very few novels.

He took enormous pains with everything he did. Having once been hurt by a critical letter from a member of the public, he arranged for a friend to drive him to the writer's address, where he made notes, before being driven back to London. He then wrote an excoriating reply to the man, containing criticisms of his house and garden.

Williams himself lived alone in a spartan, unwelcoming flat. He had, like Sherlock Holmes, a 'catlike love of personal cleanliness', and talking to Russell Harty in 1974 said he was revolted by 'sludge' under the soap. He sealed his cooker with cellophane to keep it clean and was very sensitive to mess and noise. Footsteps bothered him and when the occupant of the flat above disturbed him by moving about or playing music, he poured out his venom.

In a gripping interview with Owen Spencer-Thomas on BBC London, Kenneth Williams expanded on his odd traits. He said he used to cry continually in moments of great adversity and sought refuge in mirth: 'There is much in ... life that is very frightening, and every now and again you very much need the sort of safety valve that laughter supplies.'

He seemed content only when performing, and happiest, perhaps, when performing alone. He did this increasingly on chat shows, where he liked to show off his extensive and peculiar vocabulary, dropping words like 'polity' and 'otiose' with didactic precision. When asked on *Just a Minute* the archaic meaning of the word 'let' he explained without pause that it was 'the old King James word for, "stop"'.

Williams entertained very few visitors. Only those privy to his three-ring telephone code could get through, and those allowed into his flat were not permitted to use the toilet. He preferred to see his friends one, or possibly, two at a time and found it almost impossible to join in with groups. On holiday, beneath a searing Tangier sky, he refused to remove his tweed jacket and relax.

After sporadic homosexual fumblings as a young man, his sexual encounters were almost entirely with himself. In his distinctively weird delivery he told Joan Rivers in 1986 that he was, 'asexual … I should have been a monk … I'm only interested in myself and would regard any kind of "relationship" as deeply intrusive. Privacy is the most important thing in my life, and anything which invaded that would be a threat.'

Despite the threat of adults, Williams took great pleasure in children, who adored him. He told Owen Spencer-Thomas: 'There is a tremendously childish element in me', and he found children 'totally direct', explaining: 'They dress nothing up in any kind of sophistication or diplomacy.' This was true of Williams himself — he could be appallingly rude. His sometime friend Gyles Brandreth said that in the end he gave up on him after he misjudged the social mood at yet another dinner party and went too far.

Along with other traits, Kenneth Williams' extraordinary perfectionism, solitude, anxiety, strange vocal delivery, limited eye contact, sensory peculiarities, directness, narrow special interests, uncommon vocabulary, liking for sameness, loneliness, emotionality, distaste for social touch, and inability to join in, can, I believe, best be understood as indices of Asperger's syndrome.

★

I saw Jon from time to time. He had finished his post-graduate degree at the Slade and had decided to be a painter, using every moment of his spare time. He exhibited in Cork Street but to keep the wolf from the door he took a job teaching art and art history at a South London private school, where the sixth-form car park was full of Jaguars and BMWs.

Bill had submitted his PhD thesis and asked me and Lea over to his Waterloo flat. We got there mid-morning and as usual the place was full of cigarette smoke. It was untidier than usual, with foil curry containers on the floor, in the wastebasket, in the sink. The ashtrays were overflowing and there were wine bottles everywhere.

'Been having a party?' I asked. Bill said he had a cleaner who came in every week, but it seemed to be getting on top of him. He lit a cigarette and invited us to his local pub to unwind. By midday he was so unwound that we had to help him home. As we left he was too out of focus to wish us a proper goodbye. He seemed lonely. 'I'm worried about him,' said Lea on the train home.

Anthony had become a postman and was responsible for delivering to Soho and Theatreland. He started early and finished at three, when he would return to his flat to paint, or watch Ealing comedies.

Lea and I wanted to buy our own place and found a garden flat close to the station in a seaside town where the prices were lower than in the capital. Moving from our bit of London with its little shop that ground its own coffee, its Art Deco cinema, and its green spaces, was a wrench, but I had always loved the sea. And the commute to London was hardly longer than the rattly Tube journey in on the Northern Line.

Our newly converted flat had a patch of mud described in the particulars as a 'west-facing rear garden mainly laid to lawn'. We spent weekends clearing it of Victorian bottles, lumps of a corrugated air-raid shelter, and what appeared to be the skeleton of a medium-size dog. It was a terraced house so we were obliged to push the rubble through the flat in a wheelbarrow. We tore down a gnarled climber that appeared to be dead before a neighbour told us it was an old rose tree that flowered beautifully every year.

We went on holiday to the West Country and had ham and eggs in a tiny pub. Driving back to the rented cottage we bounced between the dry-stone embankments of the narrow lane. As we rounded a corner an owl took off from a post, spreading its wings in the headlights. We were miles from anyone but in the silence of the night a strange noise woke us. Out in the black someone was coughing. I sat up, every nerve alert, my catastrophising mind imagining a swarthy Thuggee squeezing through the kitchen window, strangling cloth between his teeth.

In the morning we flung open the curtains. The sky was blue and there was nothing to see for miles: only the thirsty meadows and a sprinkling of sheep. As we scanned the landscape one of the flock began producing a repetitive rasping cough. It bore none of its nocturnal menace.

★

On Monday nights I would visit the Magic Circle, tucked away in a Bloomsbury side street. Close-up magic is an ideal concern for a mechanically adept but socially inept creative person. When an

Asperger performs a close-up trick, he holds all the cards: an apt metaphor. There are no surprises for him. He is in charge. He alone knows what is going to happen next, and for once it is not him but everybody else who is taken by surprise by the unpredictable turn of events. This reversal of the social roles can be very satisfying for an autistic person, who is so often the one who feels at sea in social assignments.

On my first night at the Circle I was introduced to a magician called Terry. He was a naturalistic technician of the highest water and a wonderfully entertaining performer. Whatever he did he did superbly. After I had known him for a while I heard him suddenly play the piano one night, and was astonished by his technique and artistry. Whatever he did he had taught himself. My Aspergic desire for the highest quality in everything was rewarded just by knowing Terry. Others didn't know what I was on about, yet as Sherlock Holmes observed: 'Mediocrity knows nothing higher than itself; but talent instantly recognises genius.'

I noticed that the members of the Magic Circle were quite often as odd as me. The British mentalist Derren Brown has said that, 'magic does seem to appeal to creative and often quite isolated [people]'. I watched them around me at the club, performing for guests or delivering monologues to each other on the minutiae of their special interest. There is, I now realise, a pinch of autism in many of them. The best are wonderful entertainers; the worst are inward-looking bores. How interesting that sleight-of-hand magic is an enterprise enjoyed almost exclusively by boys and men.

★

The good thing about my publisher–boss was that after showing me the editorial ropes he left me to my own devices. As well as the mechanics and structure of English I became increasingly interested in the production side of publishing, so as well as my editorial responsibilities I organised the switchover from paper-and-paste and hot-metal printing to computer-assisted design and manufacture. I learned while I earned.

Though the boss led with a light rein, something was amiss. One day he called me over. 'You see all these unopened letters,' he said. 'This is what I do with them.' He lifted the front of his desk and a mountain of paperwork slid onto the floor, where he began pushing it into several wastepaper baskets. For a moment I thought he was joking, but he wasn't.

A week later I walked into the office to find him holding his head in his hands. 'It's the tree in my garden,' he said, giving me a haunted look. 'It's growing. What am I going to do ...?' He was not really addressing me; he sounded frankly mad.

★

A national newspaper was running a column featuring obscure and arcane questions from readers, to which other readers sent in serious or funny replies. The questions varied from, 'Are floppy disks corrupted by being placed near the floor on tube trains?' to 'Why is water wet?'

I couldn't resist it and over the next few years I sent in numerous carefully considered and artfully composed replies. All were entirely bogus, some ludicrously so. To have a letter published you needed to sound authoritative and be sufficiently detailed, brief, and quirky. It was also important to use the right sort of address and the right pseudonym. My favourite pen name, of many, was, Anan Abegnaro, who I made sound like an African academic, though it was really just, 'orange banana' backwards. These spoof letters took up quite a bit of my spare time and were, I suppose, my latest special interest. It was deeply pleasing to fool editor and reader alike. Almost all of my contributions were published, first in the paper and then in a series of books. Nowadays, owing to the instant checkability of everything via the Web, this would be so much less likely to succeed without even more care and preparation. But it could be done …

★

Over my time at the Pimlico publishers I got to know the area well. One day, walking in Longmoore Street, I noticed a faded painted notice on the yellow brickwork. 'PUBLIC SHELTERS IN VAULTS UNDER PAVEMENTS IN THIS STREET' it said in white capitals on a black square. There were more in Lord North Street near the river, and in Brook Street, Mayfair. These were wartime signs showing the location of makeshift bomb shelters. Their functional lettering had a great beauty and I went in search of others in St James's, Deptford, and Bermondsey. None had the allure of the Westminster signs.

One pleasant evening, Lea and I were sitting on the lawn where long ago the patch of mud and dog bones had been. The kitchen phone rang. It was Bill's mother, a wonderfully old-fashioned middle-class English lady.

'Tom, you're ex-directory, I've been trying to get hold of you.' I knew at once what she was going to say. 'Bill died last week. He was staying with friends and they couldn't wake him. I've got him here now. He looks asleep.'

I could see the picture of Bill, laid out on the mahogany table of his mother's Reigate mansion, his beard brushed — for once.

'I don't know what to say,' I said.

'Nobody does,' she replied with admirable stiff upper lip. 'I shan't say more because I'm finding it difficult to keep my emotions in check.'

She was a remarkable example of that distinctive type, of which there remain very few: the upright English matron.

We went to the funeral with Anthony.

'Was it a heart attack?' he asked.

'Too much beer, too many fags, and a diet too rich in curries,' I guessed.

At the wake, a large dog had defecated on the lawn. I felt awkward, standing there clutching a cucumber sandwich, unable to talk to anyone. Lea smoothed a few introductions and oiled the gears all round. Unlike me, she inspires confidence in people, and, being the least autistic person I have ever met, has become my praetorian guard in social situations.

The best partners for Aspergers seem to be either people like themselves — who share the same behavioural constitution and similar emotional needs — or stark complementary opposites. My inward-looking personality and Lea's outward-looking one augmented each other.

'Let's go to the pub,' said Anthony.'

'It's a shame Bill's not here,' I said. 'He'd like a pint now.'

★

Our son Jake was born. He was small and monkey-like. We needed more space so we let our flat and took a house further up the road. One day I saw a young woman picking rosemary from the bush in our garden. She rang the bell. 'Hello,' she smiled. 'I live on the corner. Celia who was here before you always let me take some rosemary when I needed it.'

'Help yourself,' I said. She had put me in the position where I could hardly refuse.

'Where's your wife?' she asked, coming into the sitting room.

'Taken the baby for a walk.'

She held the rosemary to my nose. 'It's got a lovely perfume,' she said. I sniffed the herb and as I did so she picked a thread from my sleeve. We discussed the weather, the neighbours, and her boyfriend.

'Celia went to a wife swapping party,' she said suddenly, giving me a quirky smile that I didn't understand.

'My uncle went to one of those and ended up with his own wife,' I said, repeating a joke I had heard in 1975. I didn't have a clue what was going on.

The young woman's smile vanished. I knew something had gone wrong, but I wasn't sure what. She looked at me coldly for a moment, a flicker of contempt in her eye, before striking me down with a brusque smile and letting herself out.

Life ticked over. We watered the garden, read books, and went to the shops in our unreliable Mini. Young Jake grew. My handlebar moustache grew, and was still unfashionable. Street urchins would throw orange peel and contumely in my direction as I passed. Three hundred and fifty years ago Samuel Pepys noted the same 'absurd nature of Englishmen, that cannot forbear laughing and jeering at every thing that looks strange'. Lea took a media job in government. I stayed where I was. Sameness!

A couple moved in next door. The man put his head through the hedge. 'Hello,' he said. 'Fancy a pint?' This was Mervyn, who was to become my staunch drinking companion over the next quarter of a century. He is positive, puts up with my strangeness, and keeps in touch even though we now live in different towns. He is one of my 'normal' friends, and is also happy to talk to me about typography or road signs.

One evening, he knocked on the door. 'Do you want this?' he asked, flourishing a lobster. 'The girls are in tears because I said I was going to drop it in boiling water.' The lobster gesticulated in slow motion, its claws held shut by elastic bands. I told him I didn't want to watch this handsome insect struggle and scream as it died in the pan.

'We'll stab it,' said Mervyn. 'Have you got a sharp knife?' He put the lobster on the kitchen floor and I held it. Then he sank the knife in where he said it was supposed to go. Young Jake was fascinated.

★

The boss was becoming increasingly peculiar. His desk was now a garbage heap of unanswered letters and he wandered the corridors aimlessly, fretting about the finances and the tree in his garden. He turned to me one day with a frown: 'If God made everything,' he reflected, 'who made God?' This seemed to me one of the basic questions one ought to have come to a conclusion about before taking up a lifelong career in religious publishing. He couldn't go on and retired early, being replaced by a new, prematurely bald man of emetic piety.

Of all my bosses, the bald man was the only one who never noticed how uncomfortable I felt around other people, and made no effort to accommodate my quirkiness. The neuroticism of his educated, more congenial predecessor was replaced by an offensive tactlessness. He thought it absurd that I drove a Mini, and frequently told me so.

He was unencumbered by clue and ruled the office by fiat, which struck me as not only inefficient but wrong. After I began querying his arbitrary decrees on technical matters, about which I knew more than he did, he told me, 'You have a problem with authority.' As with much of his peevish analysis this was false. It is true that, like many Aspergers, I resist 'mere' authority, whereby people are given orders without appeal to the tribunal of reason, though I do accept that a competent mother, for example, must rule on bedtimes and stop her child running into the road. But authority should generally be viewed with great suspicion and challenged at every point. We call this attitude rational vigilance, not 'a problem with authority'. My real 'problem', of course, was not with authority, but with the bald man. 'He's all piss and wind,' said a colleague, 'like the barber's cat.'

At a Tube station late one evening I was waiting for a train to come up on the indicator board when I spotted a blind man with a white cane feeling his way along the empty platform. He was gently drifting to the left and heading unwittingly for the platform edge. All at once his stick dropped into the abyss and he gesticulated wildly backwards, recovering himself just in time as a white-faced member of staff ran to his aid.

This minor cabaret having finished, I absently examined the Tube map on the wall. Over the years this archetype of good design has sunk deep into my psyche and I am alert to every change or addition. The best I applaud but the worst infuriate me.

Despite all the tinkering over the years the Underground map has survived essentially intact for nearly eight decades. It was the creation of a diagram nerd named Harry Beck, who in 1933 was encouraged by his dynamic boss Frank Pick to improve the bewildering traditional Tube map: a wormery of coloured lines confusingly superimposed on the surface topography of London's streets.

Beck developed a revolutionary de-cluttered map of the Tube system. Its secret was that it was a map in name only. Dispensing with slavish geographical accuracy, he lifted the Tube lines from their serpentine meanderings, and, like an electrician drawing a circuit board, repositioned them horizontally, vertically, or at an angle of forty-five degrees on a plain white background. Gone was the ghastly snarl of wandering Tube lines, and in its place was a plain rule-governed schematic showing just the lines. Beck equalised the spaces between stations, pulling outlying stops in towards the centre, and though he greatly distorted the geography of London the new diagram was an instantaneous hit with passengers, who, being in a tunnel, didn't care about geographic considerations such as exactly how far A was from B. Simple diagrammatic clarity overruled sprawling topographical exactitude and the new Tube map soon became a model of clear information design — an unbeatable template for transport diagrams around the world. Nowadays its popularity also makes it an attractive motif for tourist T-shirts, mugs, and other profitable tat.

★

I had been at the publisher's too long and I heard that an international accountancy firm wanted someone to manage their publications. Here was a job that would make use of all my editorial, production, design, and technical skills, and pay me better. I sent them a letter and was asked to an interview.

I understood now that a job interview was a game that, once you knew the rules, could be played to your advantage. So I went to a bookshop, where the 'business', 'self-help', and 'personal growth' sections had expanded hugely, and bought a how-to-succeed-in-interviews book. It was a treasure trove of likely questions and rules of behaviour for the game. The eye-opening instructions told me to: 1) Prepare a thirty-word statement that sublimated my story persuasively, 2) Give affirmative answers to every question: it was forbidden to drop below the zero line. If asked a question such as, 'Why did you fail?' I should have up my sleeve a positive response. For example: 'Even the best cricketer is sometimes bowled out' or 'I learnt a lot from that valuable experience'. Persuasive language, restricted hand and arm movement, and a high smile-rate were, apparently, the keys to success.

The idea that you could, or should, prepare for an interview in quite this way had never crossed my mind, and it seemed intrinsically dishonest. Perhaps it was the reason that the brash snake-oil salesmen often landed the jobs, leaving their more technically able but less calculating competitors in the dust.

I practised, as instructed, got a good haircut, as instructed, polished my shoes, as instructed, and went for the interview at an office near St Paul's Cathedral. I kept well above the zero line with my prepared answers. It was outrageous flimflam but I got the job and was put in the communications team.

The department was led by a grouse-shooting and cuff-shooting partner of the firm: a double-breasted, chalk-stripe ex-newspaperman whose alloy of urbanity and Fleet Street scar tissue enabled him to charm journalists away from the deadliest question. Technology, though, was beyond him and it was rumoured that he had once used correction fluid to paint out a typo on his computer screen. His secretary printed off all his incoming emails, which he would read before leaving for his daily eleven o'clock 'meeting' outside the office, returning at three, smelling of beer.

The accountancy firm was full of high flyers: very intelligent people who really kept me on my toes. Yet their brainpower was of a constrained type. They were extremely well informed, and really knew numbers, but they didn't make connections in the way I did. One very bright guy refused to hold a meeting in room thirteen, because he was superstitious. How intelligent is that? I wondered.

They were the most conscientious people I have ever worked with, and the industrious atmosphere was good for my anxiety. If you said to someone, 'Can you let me have those notes by nine o'clock on Tuesday?' you could then forget it. You didn't have to ask twice. At five to nine on Tuesday they would be dropped on your desk.

As well as dealing with the firm's publications, of which there were many, I had to edit the senior partner's internal newsletter. This was always larded with metaphors from sport and military conflict: it was all about *winning*. Being an aggressive, competitive alpha male of the usual kind, and chairman of his own appreciation society, the senior partner took good care to dominate everyone, from the prospective alpha males who circled him, biding their time, to his secretary. I was no exception and he used to make me wait on a low chair in his office while he conducted deliberately trivial phone calls standing at his tank-sized desk. It was fascinating to observe.

The year 2000 was approaching and all the talk was of the 'new millennium'. In my Aspergery way I argued that as there was no year 0 the current millennium would not end until 31 December 2000, making 1 January 2001 the proper start of the new millennium. I soon gave up, having learnt not to go on uselessly about matters of linguistic or scientific importance that are of no social use to people.

The 'millennium bug' was said to be a thing. There were

forecasts of dire aftershocks as a result of computers being unable to tell the difference between 2000 and 1900. Systems would crash, law firms, banks, and water companies would seize up, and electricity grids would run out of juice. The firm had decided to produce a magazine setting out the wonderful ways in which it could protect clients from the cataclysm that might destroy them at one second past midnight on 31 December 1999. As I suggested ideas for the magazine's cover, a tall, dark-haired young woman approached and interrupted me with a grammar query.

'Is it "The committee *is* meeting" or "The committee *are* meeting"?' she demanded. I explained that collective nouns could be singular or plural, depending whether one was referring to their individual members or the whole group.

'In your example, either form of words will be okay,' I said. 'But be careful, because, though you can say "The committee nodded their heads" or "The committee was smaller when I sat on it", you cannot say "The committee nodded its head" or "The committee were smaller when I sat on them."'

This seemed to annoy the tall, dark-haired, young woman. She gave an impatient snort, and, swivelling on her axis, pushed off with her nose in the air. 'What a very annoying person,' I thought.

The millennium arrived with none of the predicted disasters, though much lucrative consulting business had been done. I had changed seats and found myself sitting near the annoying, tall, dark-haired, young woman, who fired hostile glances in my direction. After a week she was put in the empty chair beside me. 'Great!' I thought. 'Fantastic! I'm stuck next to this humourless cow for the foreseeable future.'

But once again I had made a mistake. Her name was Josephine and she turned out to be a hilarious, kind, intelligent, and generous person, though she would go for the jugular if she thought someone was behaving badly. When it comes to friends, Aspergers are harpoon fishers rather than net fishers. We target people. Josephine understood me and was another dose of energetic affirmation in my life. She was patient, waving away my peculiarities. 'You are very hard on yourself,' she told me.

Now and again we would wander down Amen Court, Sermon Lane, or Paternoster Row, ancient alleys with names that doffed their caps to the hegemony of the Church, while beneath our feet the unremarked Roman bones of an earlier imperium lay at rest. Or we might visit Dr Johnson's house or have a drink in Arthur Conan Doyle's watering hole, Ye Olde Cheshire Cheese, both of which were nearby. Josephine seemed able to drink any amount of malt whisky without becoming noticeably plastered. We have been friends now for more than two decades.

At about this time, the UK government introduced new regulations for the design of the letters used on vehicle number plates. Over the preceding decade there had been an increasing laxity in what was being allowed, which offended my Aspergic respect for rules, coherent systems, and also high quality design. The new system was brilliant and soon became one of my special interests.

Like the Snellen eye-test characters and the Calvert and Kinneir typographic characters, the newly designed number plate characters took into account the special conditions that affected their legibility in the real world. Novel features had been introduced to increase clear identifiability. The letters have no serifs, except for just two, the B and the D. I wondered about this until I realised that the serifs, which otherwise add complexity where simplicity is required, prevent those two letters being mistaken at a distance, at night, or in mist, for the figures 8 and 0. Like Calvert and Kinneir's letterforms, the new numberplate characters had other legibility-improving touches, such as the straightening of the ends of diagonals on the K, X, and Y, and the oblique cutting of curved terminals on the C, G, J, and S. I tried to interest others in all this but was met with blank stares. It was fifteen years before that I met another number plate enthusiast. He told me he belonged to a club for the number plate cognoscenti, and was writing a book on the subject. He also mentioned that he had Asperger's syndrome. I was unsurprised.

I continued to travel to work from the south coast — not by road but by rail. One chilly morning a train was slowly pulling out of the station. As it did so a man holding a prayer book got down from the platform and put himself gently under the wheels. There was a lot of shouting as he was slowly mangled. An expressionless man next to me on the platform took a steady drag on his cigarette, blowing blue smoke into the air. I was equally expressionless.

Every morning I would surreptitiously study in the scratched glass the reflections of my fellow commuters. There was a bookish grey-haired couple who I dubbed Doctor and Professor Tramadol. They had jobs, I supposed, in a concrete polytechnic and were probably bad at shuffling cards.

Work was busy and the accountants bright and hardworking, but after eighteen months their tendency to rigid thought had become tiresome. They admired the material results of my work, for I am conscientious, and insist on high quality. But though I am a concrete thinker my mind tends to roam playfully, which made them suspicious of my methods. I was, once again, a fish out of water, and I decided to leave.

I found myself a job with a magazine publishing company, the proprietor of which was, implausibly, an art historian and Oxford don. With the grand title of Managing Editor I was charged with relaunching one of his undernourished journals and turning it into a successful magazine. From my City foxhole this had looked like an exciting idea, but I was to be no less a square peg than before, and had I paused I might have spotted that this was the latest in a series of round holes. I would have to take orders from the managing director and give orders to a team of writers, neither of which had I ever been very good at. Nonetheless I said yes. I told Josephine I was going. 'Don't leave me here!' she cried.

On my last day they arranged a small leaving presentation, at which I cringed. Then I went down in the lift and crossed the vestibule's terrazzo floor for the final time. As I passed through the revolving door out into the fresh air of Fleet Street the sun was bouncing off the cement of the surrounding offices. Beside a pillar-box a bird was worrying a discarded sausage and at an open window a man in shirtsleeves was fiddling with a loudhailer. Catching my eye he put the thing to his lips.

'Good afternoon!' he announced. People looked round.

'That's nice and loud,' I shouted back. We both laughed. I was forty-one and my hair was starting to recede.

Chapter 6:
Changed priorities ahead

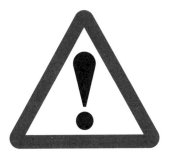

**The highest forms of understanding we can achieve
are laughter and human compassion.**

RICHARD FEYNMAN

We had moved into a black-and-white 1920s house near a park by some allotments popular with arsonists. Every now and again the crackle and roar of a torched shed would awaken us, its orange light flickering over the shadow of the bedroom wall. When we redid the bathroom the builders found a Woodbine cigarette box under the floorboards: the dusty packet that now stands on my bookcase, next to my bust of William Blake. The house by the park was a good place for my young son to grow up but it was twenty minutes further from the railway station.

The magazine publisher's new offices were not in the middle of London, as I'd been told, but in an out-of-the-way, inconvenient, and ugly part of town close to the home of the managing director. The journey to work was an Icelandic Saga and worries about the rush-hour journey, and all those people, were disturbing my sleep. I decided to travel earlier.

Rising at four fifteen I would take a bleary cab to my local station, where I would catch a train to London. I would then take two Underground trains, followed rain or shine by a brisk fifteen-minute walk up a hill to the office, sinking down at my desk two-and-a-half hours after slamming my first train door. After a day of troubles I would be away by seven to redo the journey in reverse, getting home at nine-thirtyish, in time for some cold leftovers and three fingers of Lagavulin. It was an Asperger's nightmare: crowds, hubbub, misapprehension, and unexpected change. At the weekend I would fall asleep on the sofa. Perhaps a more normal person might have said, 'Hang on a second; why are you doing this?'

The job itself played to many of my technical skills, but it was highly demanding and in my first eighteen months I was running up and down stairs from finance meeting (quite beyond me) to editorial meeting to production meeting, while trying, first, to get the magazine redesigned and relaunched, and, then, written and published. Everything was always urgent and my low tolerance of incompetence, poor quality, and delay was winding me up like a drumming monkey.

The managing director was young, brisk, confident, ill informed, and incurious. When I announced that I had decided to headline a boring feature on carpets 'THE ROAD TO UNDERLAY' everyone laughed. 'I don't get it,' she said. She drove a BMW, the roof of which could be wound down, and she liked to let you know that it had air conditioning — then still an exclusive extra. Management speak was another of her preoccupations and she was an 'early adopter' of such neologisms as 'enabling' and 'leveraging', keen too on 'monetising deliverables' and 're-envisioneering synergistic value-added paradigms going forward'. She made no allowance for my eccentricities.

When she told me quietly that she was prepared to be less than truthful about a private meeting with a difficult member of staff who was threatening her with an employment tribunal I was shocked.

'There were only two of us in that room,' she remarked coolly. 'I can say what I like.'

'But that's dishonest,' I objected.

'Honesty is very important to you, isn't it?' she said, eyeing me curiously, as if I had just said that I was compelled to take my temperature every hour.

As well as everything else, I was obliged to deal — not very well — with a small team of journalists. Beyond the technicalities of their writing I was not very good at managing them. Sorting out who had called who a fat cow and untangling their requests for simultaneous holidays took up more time than it ought to have done. I tried my best but was hampered by my quiet inwardness and ham-fisted social flubbing.

My best writer, Davit, was a waspish gay American with body odour. He was having trouble with a headline for a story about a hospital that had been converted into an estate of flats and houses.

'What about, "Bedside Manor"?' I said.

'Brilliant every time!' said Davit.

'A knack; that's all.'

One day, having taken a lungful of Davit's shirt effluvium full in the chest, the managing director asked me to tell him to bathe. A colleague once described me as 'pathologically autonomous', and disliking giving orders as much as taking them I bridled. To be completely free it is not only necessary to avoid being a slave it is also necessary to avoid becoming a master.

'I am now *instructing* you to tell him,' the boss insisted pompously.

Resisting authority and conformity of every kind, Aspergers tend to plough their own quirky furrow, baulking at the standard. Their defining characteristic is that they are not standard, and their leaning towards critical objection to mere authority makes conflict almost inevitable, particularly if those in charge of them lack insight into their peculiar difficulties.

I had a lot in common with the strange members of the IT department, who, to a man, I now realise, were autistic. Though their rude communication style irritated some people, I got on well with them. One had an obsession with cooking and another spent his weekends dressing up in chain mail and parading in medieval reenactments. In his remaining spare time he was a lutenist of repute. He had also invented some sort of software and people wrote articles about him in technical journals.

The finance director was a polished graduate, whose public-school voice was used for the answering machine message. He favoured jumbo cords and ate greasy-spoon breakfasts with an ironic smile. One day he gave me a ride to the station on the back of his motorbike. 'Hold on to me!' he yelled as we rounded a sharp bend, but I hated to touch him. He told me about an old school friend who was a political aide for a very famous English politician and organised sex parties in smart Chelsea houses in his spare time. 'The first one you go to is a bit strange,' Jumbo Cords told me. 'You climb these marble steps and inside everyone is sitting around drinking and chatting. It's a bit tense — you all know why you're there — then after a bit it suddenly all starts happening.' The thought of all those people made me shudder.

Someone from the sales department buzzed my phone.

'I've got a customer on the line,' she said. 'He's furious about something or other. He's got a really really strong accent.'

I told her to put him through.

'Good afternoon, Sir,' I said. 'How can I help?'

'You have fucked me!' he announced. His blunt claim took me aback, and though I tried to get to the bottom of his complaint he kept repeating his statement in a guttural accent.

'What would you like me to do?' I asked. I had the feeling that there must be more to this than met the ear.

'You have *fucked* me!' he said again. Though emphatic, he was, I realised, not angry. He was trying to explain something. All at once the penny dropped.

'Oh, I see,' I said. 'We've *faxed* you, have we?'

'Yes. Yes.'

He was delighted that someone had finally understood. I dealt with his query and explained things to the sales department. They laughed immoderately, and the cheerful sales director, who lived in a country house with a flooded cellar full of floating wine bottles, invited me out for a kebab. Waving at the elephant's leg on a stick rotating in front of the heat he said: 'Don't eat that stuff. I know what's in it.'

★

I went to interview the actor Simon Callow at his house not far from the flat over the knocking shop, where I had lived with Alice.

295

Except for a hideous new supermarket, the area was unchanged. One side of a street would be full of smart professionals in skinny white houses, the opposite side a jumble of multi-occupancy dwellings whose peeling exteriors were pocked with satellite dishes and entryphone boxes. Poverty clings to stucco. Under the streaked render of one such building I saw a young couple embracing in a mossy doorway. The man's trousers were round his ankles.

I stopped at the pedestrian crossing by the Tube. Ever since a scare with a sports car I no longer dashed across but waited for the green man. As I stood there I perused a beautiful Kinneir/Calvert traffic sign pointing to Crouch End, Hampstead, and Highgate. Jock Kinneir believed that consistency in design was the visual equivalent of grammar in language, and described direction signs as 'vital as a drop of oil in an engine, without which the moving parts would seize up'. On both counts he was right, and the signs that he and Calvert designed prove it.

Simon Callow's house was a beautiful early Victorian cube of yellow brick, adorned with pilasters and volutes. He let me in out of the pouring rain and showed me into what was either a large sitting room or a very large study. I wasn't sure because, although there was a sofa, stalagmites of books were growing up from most of the floor. On the wall, a mannerist portrait of a bare-chested boy and the huge face of Oscar Wilde looked down at us. 'My place is absolutely overflowing — to an alarming degree,' Callow apologised, clearing a pile from a chair. Then, more severely, 'I can only give you half an hour.' He strode over to a telephone and dialled a number, ordering a cab for half an hour's time and making quite a performance of it.

He had written a book about *The Night of the Hunter*, a film directed by Charles Laughton, which happened to be a favourite of mine. As he warmed to his theme, continually pouring tea from a gigantic pot, we began to get on rather well. This was, and is, my preferred way to meet new people. Two of us together in a quiet well-lit room; a narrow subject matter known to me beforehand; a definite span of time during which to talk; and no chat. Like a television or radio interview, this was a facsimile conversation with its own reassuring rules. I found I was as relaxed in the question-asking role as in the question-answering one.

I have always been interested in cinema so the interview turned into a nerds' discussion. After a while I noticed that I had overstayed my half hour by twenty minutes. Callow saw me out, down the wet steps. Oddly enough the taxi he had ordered hadn't arrived.

As I walked to the station I reflected that, though I love cinema, I often get the people of the drama mixed up. I tag them by their glasses, or clothes, but a film featuring two moustachioed men in raincoats or two women with shoulder-length hair will do for me. 'Is that the man who shot the other man with the pens in his pocket?' I might ask Lea.

'No,' she will say. 'It's his father.'

Once I've got them visually sorted out I can still be confused by what they are doing.

'Why is she crying?' I recently asked as we watched a film.

'Because she loves him but she realises that he doesn't love her,' Lea explained.

The mechanical details are of more interest to me than the characters, and I am always particularly on the lookout for snow-and-ice effects. This began when, as a boy, I saw the 1930 Laurel and Hardy film *Below Zero*. Shot outside in the balmy California sun, the cold-weather effects were a mixture of crude and subtle. Ice cream was used for snowballs, leaving a giveaway oily white trail down Ollie's face, but the thick ice through which Stan falls was more convincing. I was puzzled how they did it until years later I learned that it was wax. Other highly persuasive snow-and-ice effects have, over the years, been created with cotton wool, washing powder, salt, ash, shredded plastic, baking soda and tiny acrylic spheres known as 'microballoons', and, for snow trodden underfoot, particles of paper compressed with water. Orson Welles' *Citizen Kane*, made just eleven years after *Below Zero*, contains much better snow effects. For *The Magnificent Ambersons* (1942) Welles shot some superb snow scenes in a Los Angeles icehouse: the first time that characters' breath had been visible on the cold air. *Those Magnificent Men in Their Flying Machines* (1965) used an old long-shot favourite: gallons of industrial foam, though the wind blew it around very unconvincingly in huge globs. *Murder on the Orient Express* (1974) used the same material much better, augmenting it with wonderful creaking-snow sound effects.

I have yet to meet another person who shares my special interest in snow effects, or my preoccupation with the design of the special characters used on UK number plates, or my enthusiasm for the wonderful shapes-disguised-as-letters that appear on the Snellen eye-test chart. Odd preoccupations, I now realise.

Although I do not expect everyone to share my strange interests, some people do 'get me'. Being visually sophisticated and culturally developed, my friend Mervyn is one of those with an eye for the technicalities that so absorb me. One day as we drove along a main road towards a pub lunch something caught my eye.

'Hang on,' I said. 'These road signs look different.'

The car slowed as we approached a junction and I was able to scrutinise a big sign near the slip road. While remaining essentially the same as the signs I was used to it seemed to have been smoothed and polished. I saw that instead of being manufactured from separate bits of material glued down in place it was now of a single piece. I realised what had happened.

'They've digitised them,' I said.

Mervyn peered over his sunglasses. 'You're right,' he said. 'What do you think?'

'It works,' I said. 'I like them.'

I was amazed. The new signs resembled a set of much-loved cut crystal glasses that had been replaced overnight with an identical set, but one with a higher lead content: sharper, brighter, and more refractive. I was delighted.

*

The journeys to and from work were taking it out of me. Coming home late one night I was buttonholed on the station steps by a bearded person wearing a poncho and holding a smashed-up guitar. 'If you're just getting back from work,' he said, 'you're an idiot.' I hadn't the strength to kick him, and to be fair he had a point. I walked the twenty minutes back to the house and sat on the bottom stair to take off my shoes. 'This is insane,' I said to Lea. 'I don't know how much more I can take.'

I had been mulling over an idea. I remembered the great pleasure I'd had in the eighties writing spoof letters to the paper and the glee with which I had read Joe Orton's Edna Welthorpe letters. I also recalled Gerard Hoffnung's spoof letters supposedly from Tyrolean hoteliers struggling with poor English: 'Do not concern yourself that I am not too good in bath; I am superb in bed.' Could I write some funny letters in a similar vein, using language mix-ups? And could I come up with a plausible character who always got the wrong end of the stick? I thought I could, and I had an idea how it might be done.

★

One day the MD collared me in the corridor, objecting to the noun 'nitty-gritty' in a piece I had okayed. 'It's racist,' she scolded. 'It's about the nits on slaves. Didn't you know?' She seemed very pleased with herself, but I was sceptical. My reference books mentioned nothing about it, so I emailed the *Oxford English Dictionary*. They explained that 'nitty-gritty' had nothing to do with slaves, and that 'nitty-' was most probably a meaningless rhyme attached to 'gritty' after the fact. Etymology being one of my interests, I was fascinated. I was also vindicated. I copied the email to the MD — a mistake, as detail, and being wrong, was not her thing.

She called me into her office, seeming peeved. 'As the managing editor you are doing too much editing and not enough managing,' she said. Along with my mad commute, this latest of her world-turned-upside-down pronouncements was a signal that it was time to go. I had worked hard but once again my relationships with people, including the MD, had not developed as they might have done. Everything everyone else enjoyed I hated. Everything I enjoyed everyone else found peculiar or infantile. I handed in my notice. 'What are you going to do?' asked the sales director, polishing his glasses. I told him I was going to write a book. 'Christ!' he said.

The boss informed me that as a farewell she would be taking me out to eat some food with a lot of the office people. She told us to meet her in one of her favourite bars but she went to the wrong place and left us waiting. What a Freudian would make of that I don't know. When she finally turned up she demanded that a big table be pulled into place for us all to sit around and there was an excruciating fuss as waiters rearranged the furniture. I explained that this was not what I wanted but she couldn't hear me. However, the irresistible force had met the immovable object: I picked up my briefcase and left my own leaving party, without so much as a Pan Am smile.

Someone had asked me: 'How are you going to write at home? You'll just be lounging around in a silk dressing gown drinking pink gins,' but I found that the solitary life of the writer suited me, and my nitpicking and self-criticism were apt for the maintenance of quality. I had dug around in my files and found a spoof letter I had written fifteen years earlier, when Lea and I had been living in the flat opposite the wood. It was by one of my alter egos, Tomas Santos, a young man of indeterminate nationality who was studying at a language college on the South Coast. His English was terrible, but he was blessed with a gift for the inspired guess, though the misunderstandings and double entendres were many and rude. This was the character I had decided to develop for my book of letters.

The mechanics of language were meat and drink to me, but if I were to pull off this trick I would need to pick my targets carefully. So I made a list. There was a scattering of people I admired, but most were Establishment figures that I hoped to poke fun at or just inconvenience, using as my weapons Tomas Santos and his mangled English.

Over the next year Tomas wrote letters in tortured English to hundreds of people. He asked the Master of the Rolls for 'two cheese and tomato on brown, with poopy seeds'. He wrote to the Lord Archbishop of Armagh, wondering why the Church was led by a 'primate' and advising him not to eat too many bananas, and to the Queen at Buckingham Palace, 'Near the roundabout', asking for a 'singed photograph' (a recurring motif). Most people replied, some, like Sir George Martin and Noam Chomsky, with respect and charm, others with ludicrous pomposity. I used to run downstairs in the morning to see what had arrived and got the most fun from the sniffy ones. Sheltering behind the façade of Tomas gave me a wonderful sense of irresponsible freedom, which I found lacking in ordinary life.

Tomas Santos wrote to the philosopher Mary Warnock, who had intrigued me when she had once bought dinner for my old friend Jon and me after he had exhibited some paintings in a picture gallery with which she had a slight connection. She struck me then as delightfully odd, but it was not till recently that I discovered that she had had an autistic brother, and that her unusual mother had been an independent-thinking eccentric who wore strange clothes and walked with splayed feet — a physical characteristic of note in autistic people. I now understand Lady Warnock's charming oddity in a new way. In Tomas' letter to her he asked for her views on a principal of contemporary philosophy, the subject known as 'causality'. She replied, pointing out that, unfortunately, he had got the wrong idea: 'I fear you mistook CAUSALITY for CASUALTY — a hospital soap opera,' she said. I enjoyed the crash of gears that Tomas often produced by his 'misunderstandings', but was this not a strange way to communicate with people, and a strange way to enjoy oneself?

After a year or so I had amassed box files of letters and replies. It was time to try to get published. I had been told that this was best done through an agent but that if I thought getting a publisher would be hard, getting an agent would be harder. For all that, I did what you are supposed to do and bought a copy of the *Writers' and Artists' Yearbook*, circling some of those agencies which said they handled humour. Instead of a standard letter I sent each a Tomas Santos letter. Here is an example:

Laura Morris Literary Agency

Dear Laura,

I am visiting in UK since a short time that I may study in the language college and read many the English book to speak in a well idiom.

My intensively reading incorporated some the classic, like Charles Dickens: *Oliver Twit*, L. M. Montgomery: *Anne of Green Bagels*, and Grahame Greene: *Travels With My Cunt*. I ever wished to wrote the book, but in my home land ours military leaders precluded seditious writings so I must hid them in the hole in my uncle's back passage. Now, however, it my big chance and I have the idea for the book that is 'ready to go'. This are my *Collected Correspondences* that I collected him hunderds letters in a only year. Here what some people said that my letters:

'Our sauce contains tamarinds – a tropical fruit – not tamarins, which are monkeys!'

HP FOODS

'"Primate" is an ecclesiastical term …'

ARCHBISHOP ROBERT EAMES

'I am happy to be Patron of your band, *Wind, String & Faggots*.'

TONY HAWKS

'We do not allow indoor BBQs within the Ritz Hotel.'

RITZ HOTEL

'*Very funny* letter. You should be published.'

VICTOR LEWIS-SMITH

'Obviously you need help.'

THE SAMARITANS

I anticipate to ours excitable pratnership Laura and I put the stamp for good responding manners.

Yours friend,
TOMAS SANTOS

Some agents replied, others didn't bother, despite Tomas enclosing postage. Laura Morris, the addressee of the above letter did reply, asking me to visit her, bringing everything I had ever written. 'Everything I had ever written' amounted to these letters, so I made a collection of a few of my favourites and went to see her. We talked about Sherlock Holmes, Alfred Hitchcock, painting, and writing. She thought we had a book in the offing and said she would try to find me a publisher.

Like the best agents, Laura made allowances for my foibles. She called me 'A complete original', which is a kind way to describe the idiosyncrasies that many find so disagreeable. She has been my agent, and friend, now for more than fifteen years.

Women have always been important to me, and most of my few friends are female. One day one of them gave me a book. It was by a man called Mark Haddon and its title was *The Curious Incident of the Dog in the Night-time*. I didn't like the cover or the typography but I recognised the title as a quotation from Sherlock Holmes so despite its being fiction I decided to read it. The text had been set in a sans serif typeface, which made it tiresome to read, because serifs guide the eye horizontally as you go. It was also sprinkled with careless setting mistakes. I noticed an extraneous letterspace between the words 'logic' and 'can' in line three of paragraph two on page eighty-two. All the same, I was intrigued and strangely touched by the story. I found that the interests and feelings of the main character, a boy called Christopher, tended to reflect my own: his dismay in busy railway stations; his liking for details, and patterns, and rules; his confusion when meeting new people; and his interest in Sherlock Holmes. Someone told me the character was autistic but I dismissed this on the ground that his thoughts and behaviour were not autistic: this was how everybody felt. By 'everybody', I now realise, I meant 'me'. I completely failed to make the connection.

★

Laura had had a great response from a publisher to my Tomas Santos book. But he wondered whether, before he published the letters, Tomas could first write an English phrasebook for foreigners. Like the jobless actor who is asked by a film producer 'Can you speak siSwati?' I automatically said yes.

So I got to work, writing dialogues such as *In the Restaurant*, *To Speak with Childrens*, and *To Met the Queen*. Because I now knew Tomas Santos intimately it all flowed quite easily. I called the book, *Speak Well English: an guide for aliens to successful intercourse in the correctly English mode* and when it was done I sent it off. When it came out various radio stations wanted to interview me and one asked me to do it in character. I had to improvise, which was exhilarating and terrifying at the same time, but it played to my exhibitionistic Asperger strengths. After five minutes, they asked if I could stay for half an hour. I said yes, and in that time I reduced the whole team to incapable laughter. I have never felt happier; when I came out into the street afterwards I was floating.

The publisher told a colleague he thought the book 'the funniest thing we've ever published', but the reading public were not so enthusiastic and it sold less well than hoped. It seemed that the professionals were as ignorant as anyone else about what people would and wouldn't buy; otherwise, I supposed, they would publish nothing but best sellers. You couldn't tell the reading public what they liked: they told you.

Nevertheless, being a 'published author' opened doors, and an editor called Dan, who worked for one of the big publishers, asked to meet me. Book publishing in London had long since ceased to be a club of gentlemen in superb suits reclining in smoke-filled Bloomsbury offices; Dan was based at an American-style headquarters near an uncommonly hideous flyover on the western fringe of the city. I reported to a receptionist in a foyer decorated with spiky plants in acrylic tanks full of pebbles. Looking up into the atrium I counted floor after floor of pale green frosted-glass offices. The atmosphere put me on edge. I don't know whether this was my Aspergic sensory sensitivities rebelling against the fingernails-down-blackboard interior design, or just the normal revulsion of a person with a taste for the shapes of nature and a sense of proportion.

Dan bounced into reception to meet me. I immediately took to his naughty-schoolboy energy.

'I want you to write a book,' he said.

'Oh? What book?' I asked.

'A humorous, spoofy how-to book for boys, covering every subject under the sun.'

'From how to light a fire to how to light a fart?'

'You've got it!' said Dan.

The 'target reader' was not really boys, but anybody from six-teen up who liked to laugh. I knew at once I could do it. Dan told me to go away and come up with two hundred ideas for suitable subjects, which I did. We met again a week later and I brought out my pages-long roll call of subjects, among which were flags, languages, maps, music, Morse code, rain gauges, semaphore, the Beaufort wind scale, palindromes, the manufacture of concrete, human anatomy, the Fibonacci series, gardening, orders of magni-tude, and aircraft tail insignia. Dan approved. These were subjects of interest to me and I enjoyed being funny about them. Examining the list now I notice that they are stereotypically autistic: systems all.

We were joined by a man who wanted to talk about how to market the book, with no budget.

'Right,' he said, 'first things first: who do you know?'

'Nobody,' I said. 'I am the worst connected author you will ever meet.'

211 Things a Bright Boy Can Do was brought out in good time for the Christmas shopping jamboree. On the day of publication Dan rang me. 'Do you know your book's number fifteen on the Amazon bestsellers list?' Over the next three months it climbed the rankings, peaking at number one, where it stayed for a while. Everyone, including me, was astonished. Walking down Piccadilly I saw it filling a huge bookshop window.

Everyone loves a success. A production company got in touch and wanted to use me to front a proposed television show. 'We haven't had a "mad professor" for ages,' they said. We filmed some stuff and they pitched the idea but as is so often the case nothing came of it. I was asked to appear on *Loose Ends*, and I remembered listening to the show all those years ago in the kitchen of the house opposite the woods. I could hardly believe I was now *on* it. The book was sold to many foreign countries. It did well in America, and a producer on David Letterman's famous show wanted me as an interviewee: a Big Deal. I was all ready to be flown out, when the writers went on strike and the programme was taken off the air for a couple of months. The slot gone, I missed my chance to show off in front of the biggest audience yet, but consoled myself with Steve Martin's remark that you had to do the show half a dozen times before people realised they had seen you.

211 Things became a bestseller in Germany and sold spectacularly well in France. The country where it did best per head of population was, curiously, Finland. Nobody could quite understand why. I knew that all this positive attention would go away again, which kept my feet on the ground but disabled me from enjoying it.

Still, the money meant I could now try to write for a living without the need to keep chasing the mortgage. I was attracted by the idea of the isolated author, beavering away untroubled by the stress of office chat around the water cooler. It looked like the perfect job for me, though I didn't yet understand that it was my Aspergers that really made it so suitable.

Why does anyone decide to write a book? The writing racket is about as glamorous as any other glamorous profession — that is to say, not at all glamorous. And only rarely will the money feed a family. George Orwell described writing as 'a horrible, exhausting struggle' that no one would undertake unless driven by some demon, 'whom one can neither resist nor understand'.

The author of narrative non-fiction must, as E. B. White suggested, 'take his trousers off without showing his genitals', and to be any good he or she must possess, like the genius, an infinite capacity for taking pains, which is certainly one of the Asperger's strengths. Jean Anouilh put it in a nutshell: 'The object of art is to give life a shape', and I think this best explains what is going on. The Asperger and non-Asperger writer alike can make sense on the page of all the unpredictable chaos of real life, over which they otherwise have no control.

The philosopher Søren Kierkegaard said that only when he wrote did he feel well. When I am writing, I do not feel *well*, exactly, just less anxious. Like Sherlock Holmes relieving the tension with his seven-per-cent solution of cocaine, writing is my drug. The actress and writer Emma Thompson described writers as fundamentally inconsolable, and compared writing to cutting yourself purposefully: 'It's letting something out, and suddenly you're released from this inner pain.' I agree with that absolutely.

From my first book on I continued to write sequestered in my garret. For days on end I might see nobody, and sometimes I became a bit unhinged. A few of my titles turned into bestsellers but none equalled the success of the how-to book for boys. Though I wanted to write I did not want to be well connected on the literary scene, or go to parties and press the flesh. When invited to these jamborees I go because I feel I ought to, but though I long to fit in I always manage to put my foot in it.

There was one do at which I saw Doris Lessing and a lot of other well-known faces. People chatted, smiled, mixed, worked the room, networked, struck up new contacts, while I stood alone. The quiz show host Nicholas Parsons was there I seem to recall, dressed in a blazer like a deck chair. When *Just A Minute* had been one of my special interests I would have been overawed.

There is a cliché that we are all different, but, looking round at other people at the publisher's party, they all seemed the same. I was the different one.

As I stood there in my Aspergic shutdown I became aware of a middle-aged woman heading towards me. I gripped the stem of my wine glass in apprehension.

'And what is your name?' she said, giving me a headmistress smile.

'Tom,' I said.

'Tom what?'

This annoyed me. She seemed to be fishing for information with which to place me somewhere on a scale of usefulness or importance.

'Oh, it won't mean anything to you,' I said.

She gave me a look I could not decipher, and, with the air of Narcissus gazing into the pool, announced her own name. It was one with which I was familiar. 'Well that means something to me,' I said. At once a sheet of ice formed on the woman's face and she rotated her body sharply to the right, disappearing through a doorway with what used to be called 'hauteur'. Was I behaving like Enoch Powell talking to Kingsley Amis at that party?

Later, I upset one of the marketing people by criticising the snow effects in one of her favourite films, *Bridget Jones's Diary* (2001), which contains a long shot of a snow-covered field using the old standby, a white sheet. Unhappily, I explained, the wrinkled edge doesn't reach the corner of the field, ending in a clearly visible border of summer-green grass, thus blowing the whole illusion, like a magician accidentally flashing the card he is trying to conceal in his hand. I explained that another thing that always annoyed me was falling snow in animated films that moves sideways with the camera as it pans. The marketing woman said nothing but gave me a look of scorn.

I was homed in on by a man whose face I recognised because he had presented some cookery programmes on the television. He was genial, and wanted to know what I wrote.

'Humour,' I said.

'Oh I love jokes. Tell me a joke.'

I explained that jokes are the enemy of humour but he didn't understand. I wished I were a boy again, lying alone in the dark under the twinkling Christmas tree, looking up through the boughs and savouring the perfume of the pine.

★

We moved from the house near the park into the house where I am writing this, in the old port further up the coast. When it rained I could feel the cold drops hit the bald circle of skin in the middle of my scalp, a broken tooth at the back of my mouth had been replaced by a bridge, and now and again my knee would ache wearily. It's always later than you think.

One morning, I was looking down from my office into the street, where fractal feathers were icing the bonnets of the cars, when the phone rang. It was a person from the past with the news that Katy, my girlfriend from all those years ago, had been climbing a hill when she had fallen down dead, leaving behind a child, a husband, and a career as a professor of English. I squinted back down the time-stained passage of the decades, and at the end, standing in the hoop of light, I could just make out the tiny figure of myself. Beside me was the shadow of my art teacher Miss Legge, who had been hit by the hurtling lorry. Beside her I could see Bill Bradshaw, who had died in bed in his twenties, and the dark frame of the man with the prayer book who had lain in front of the quietly departing train. But after all this time, and the battened-down loss of the years, what did I feel about Katy? Complete detachment. This special interest had faded.

★

Not far from the site of the toyshop where Bob Hoskins had got shirty with me all those years ago are the headquarters of the National Autistic Society. I had decided to visit them to find out about their hopes and plans. As usual I was forty minutes early. The weather was boiling and the pavement radiated a shimmering heat, so I dropped into an air-conditioned pub for a glass of fizzy water.

The place was cool and dark, decorated with rough planking and iron pipes set off for some reason by old ladies' lampshades. Standing against an incongruous wall of Alhambra-style geometric tiles was a black pub piano covered in white capital letters spelling out the words of some pop hit. Fixed above this tone-deaf interior a snaking mass of exposed air conditioning ceiling conduits made the place look unfinished. Two large television screens, their colours saturated to the maximum, were relaying a football match to semicircles of men in T-shirts, who groaned whenever their team fumbled the ball. All at once a goal was scored and a deafening roar went up. A baby started to cry. I knew how it felt, so I swallowed my water and left.

At the society's office I buzzed the door and was let in by a receptionist, who asked me to wait. Signs on the walls pointed to meeting rooms named after planets and behind a chair a dropped sheet of paper was sticking out at a bothersome angle.

I had arranged to see a man named Chris, who soon appeared. He took me out to a café with a twelve-foot mural of a stark-naked woman sporting breasts like balloons. I decided to sit sideways on to this distraction. We tried between us to start with some social conversation. Chris told me he was good at languages, and was just learning Icelandic. I don't recall what I said. Then we got down to business.

According to the NAS, while almost everybody has heard of autism, few really understand the condition in a meaningful way. The focus over the next few years, Chris told me, will continue to be on improving public understanding, as well as bettering autistic lives. His job is to help businesses that run theatres and other public spaces to improve their understanding of, and approach to, autistic people, who for decades have been shushed, stared at, or asked to leave.

But educating the public is like trying to push a train up a mountain. There have been some small practical improvements in recent years, with, for example, the introduction of 'autism-friendly' performances in theatres and cinemas, 'quieter hours' in supermarkets, and special training for airport staff. High-profile initiatives have included the introduction of a female character with autism into the UK television soap opera *Hollyoaks*, and *Sesame Street*'s autistic puppet, Julia. All the same, the media's wide but not very deep coverage of the condition can sometimes look like a bandwagon-jumping exercise and one could be forgiven for viewing such novelties with scepticism. Have the production companies involved, I wonder, changed their recruitment and employment practices to make things easier for autistic interviewees and workers? Have they made efforts to hire autistics to play non-autistic roles? Media executives should rend their hearts and not their garments.

But hope is a sturdy shrub and Chris is confident of a better future for autistic people. He says that the technological innovations such as smartphones are an 'anxiety lifesaver', and it is true that the development of IT and email communication has been good for autistic employees and bosses alike. If employers can make allowances they will find, perhaps for the first time, the singular contributions that a few bright and quirky corkscrew thinkers can make to success. Autistic employees are not only conscientious and industrious in their chosen work, many are also creative and extremely original. They say what they mean and mean what they say, insist on high quality, are focused, painstaking, and rule conscious, and have an extremely fine eye for detail. They are also dependable, punctual, honest, and loyal. Just so long as everyone remembers that they do not like to be bombarded with information, other people, or endless demands, and that they like to know in detail what's next, exactly where they need to be, and precisely what it is they are expected to do. A few minor adjustments and a bit of insight are all it takes from the boss.

Autistics see the world differently and feel everything more intensely than typical people, they react in unusual ways to things that most people either enjoy or take in their stride. But it is a broad spectrum and the more subtle types, like me, can be hard to spot. What people often see is an intelligent, articulate person, perhaps rather aloof, who uses grammar precisely and has a quiver full of apt words ready for his bow. How can such a person possibly be autistic? The answer is that still waters run deep, and an extensive vocabulary and good intelligence may mask real underlying problems, making it seem as though we are working at a much higher level than we are. What people often do not see in Aspergers, sometimes because it is so well camouflaged, is the confusion and dismay caused by the frequently inhospitable world: the constant self-monitoring, the anxiety, the botched social approaches and muffed relationships, the anguish, the exhaustion, the silent rage, and the deep dark cave of loneliness. Appearances can be deceptive and we can be easily overlooked, or dismissed with the term 'high functioning', as if our problems are accordingly 'mild'. It is sometimes only when an Asperger is seen in a social situation for the first time that others begin to understand just what a stranger in his own country he really is.

Autistic people die younger than average people. At the severe end of the continuum the cause is not autism itself but epilepsy, drowning, and injury. At the 'high-functioning' end it is suicide. Simon Baron-Cohen reports that two thirds of Aspergers in his clinic say they have felt suicidal, and one third have felt so bad that they have tried it. His university also found that twelve per cent of all those who deliberately end their lives are definitely or probably autistic. Ending your own life, or trying to, is not a sign that you are functioning well, it is a sign that, maybe despite appearances, you are functioning extremely poorly, that something is very seriously wrong.

Estimates vary for the prevalence of autism in the general population according to the way the numbers are counted. A figure of one in sixty-eight is commonly quoted in the USA, and more than one in a hundred in the UK. Research from King's College London and the Karolinska Institute in Stockholm shows that children are twice as likely as normal to be diagnosed with autism if they have an autistic cousin, and ten times more likely if they have a brother or sister with the condition. Having more than one autistic sibling appears to make it likelier still. Whatever the actual numbers, the family connection is clear and parents with an autistic child who are planning further children should be alert.

With the broadening of diagnoses, many people have sought to find something or someone to blame for what they mistake for a modern epidemic. But the recent discovery that there are many autistic adults struggling on through life without a diagnosis or any support makes it clear that the rise in numbers of children with autism is not a sign of a newly prevalent condition in need of a novel environmental cause.

I recently read of a research scientist, whose blushes I will spare, who published a graph showing a rise in childhood autism between 1994 and 2009 exactly matching the increased use, over that same period, of the weed killer glyphosate. Her argument looked persuasive: the climbing glyphosate line on her graph closely in sync with the line showing the increasing rate of autism. That was until I saw another graph, made by a different scientist to show how easy it is to confuse random correlation with real cause and effect. Covering a similar period, this graph showed the same very close match between the rise in autism diagnoses and the increased consumption of organic food. The increase in autism diagnoses, the rise in glyphosate use, and the growing popularity of organic food are indeed linked — but by nothing more than coincidence.

Thankfully science has now extinguished many delusions about autism, such as that refrigerator mothers or the MMR jab are the cause, though there are still pockets of credulity here and there, where unquestioning people continue to point their finger. The seemingly wilful misunderstanding of the way science works has a lot to answer for.

In *A History of Autism: conversations with the pioneers* Adam Feinstein remarks that autism remains such a complex and bewildering condition that agreeing on a definition is nearly impossible, and could be meaningless. In discussing the enduring enigma the autistic writer Donna Williams told him that we are 'merely the fools of tomorrow'.

The abolition of the term 'Asperger's syndrome' in the most recent US *Diagnostic and Statistical Manual* is part of a trend to refer to autism as a single broad neurodevelopmental condition with many different presentations. But despite this, Asperger's syndrome and classic autism are still commonly spoken of as two *distinct* things.

I heard a man talking movingly about the daily problems of looking after his adult son, who still drinks from a child's beaker; there is an ocean of difference between profound challenges like this and those of the absent-minded professor. Not only is there a range of severity along the continuum, but also a great liquorice-allsorts variety, and it seems reasonable, while accepting their obvious shared traits, to continue to recognise Asperger's syndrome and classic autism as crucially different in important ways. This is how I have treated them in this book.

Yet whether they really are truly different expressions of the same thing or two — possibly more — quite discrete complaints, is, in fact, still undecided. Families may include severely impaired autistics and Asperger types both, so there seems to be a definite genetic overlap. What this is, however, remains an ineffable mystery. In the end, all we can hope is that those who come after us might understand more.

In his book, *Neuro Tribes*, Steve Silberman encourages the idea that the autism/Asperger spectrum is part of normal 'neurodiversity', and that to remain resilient human groups need among their number people who think differently. Autism is a fundamentally different way of being, and a fundamentally useful way of being. If you doubt that take a look at the success of Silicon Valley, listen to Glenn Gould play Bach, examine the work of the staff of NASA, or watch Anthony Hopkins act.

It might be that over hundreds of thousands, or millions, of years natural selection has favoured different types of brain for different evolutionary niches, such that autistics may be showing an extreme of the ordinary variation that exists across the population. They are being selected, perhaps, for their skills at spotting patterns, and their aptitude for innovation. These are skills that help the group, even if those with these traits find the social world more of an obstacle course than more typical people. All the same, for the parent of an uncomprehending epileptic child who cannot look after herself, this might seem a high personal cost to bear for the general group advantage.

Simon Baron-Cohen's scatter plot describing the huge range of systemising and empathising traits across the whole population of typical and autistic people alike (page 104) seems to me to paint a powerfully visual, useful, and true picture of this puzzle. It is not only a scientifically rigorous chart, with obvious trends and outliers, but also a beautiful and moving snapshot of all of us human beings, with everybody you know a dot somewhere in this great flock of humanity.

When I told some friends that I had been identified as having Asperger's syndrome I got quite different responses, ranging from scepticism, to sympathy, to outrage. 'Oh, Tom,' said one of my female friends, 'I've been telling you for years you were autistic but you wouldn't listen.'

'Have you?' I said. 'I don't remember.'

'I knew you weren't listening. My nephew has autism and so does a dear friend of mine, and I could tell you were somewhere on the spectrum too.'

'How?'

'You have very high standards. You're super funny in a very witty way but you're too dry for some people to handle. They think you're rude, aloof, or awkward, and you're meticulous about your appearance — impeccable — every hair in exactly the right place, but you don't take compliments well.'

That didn't sound to me like enough for a diagnosis, but she had obviously spotted something. Just as the subtle behaviour and dress of a person who shares your political views can reveal them as members of the same club, without their having ever said anything political, the traits of Asperger's syndrome can cause a blip on the autism radar of high-functioning autistics, and those who know autistics.

Nonetheless, Sarah Hendrickx had warned me that disbelief would be the most common reaction I would get in revealing my Asperger's diagnosis to those I knew. When I told my friend Josephine she blew her top. 'What idiot told you that?!' she said. 'Why can't people just let eccentrics like you be themselves, without all this labelling crap?!' She was so cross I decided not to tell her that, despite my not really wanting to belong to a club that would stoop so low as to accept me as a member, the diagnosis had explained everything, and released me, quite miraculously, from decades of depression. When someone you like and have known for a long time tells you that he or she is a member of a secretive religious cult, or not straight but gay, or not just eccentric but autistic, it naturally pulls you up short, and you may feel protective, wounded, or incredulous. Maybe it confirms something you have suspected but didn't want verified. In any case, you have to readjust your perceptions of that person, and this is uncomfortable and can take time.

★

The first grey hairs were starting to sprout in my handlebar moustache. I had had it for thirty years, since those warm evenings on the river at the university, with Concorde flying over. For some time I had been toying with the idea of joining the Handlebar Club, a moustache society for gentlemen with 'graspable extremities', formed in 1947 in the dressing room of the entertainer Jimmy Edwards. Tracking down the club to a charming London pub I went to one of their monthly get-togethers and received a jolly welcome.

I had half expected them to be gruff veterans of the Royal Air
Force and there were indeed a couple of that sort, including one or
two of the original members. But there was also a good sprinkling
of other types. After more than a decade in the club I have realised
that Aspergers are particularly well represented among the eccentric membership: engineers, train enthusiasts, penny-farthing riders,
silent pipe-smokers, musicians, mapmakers, scientists, taxidermists,
laconic military types, and people who enjoy dressing up — as well
as a high number of social maladroits.

★

I had been invited to a large family party and had decided to
break my journey to inspect the original maquettes of Calvert and
Kinneir's road signs, held at St Bride Library off Fleet Street, close
to the office of the accounting firm where I had worked almost two
decades before. I was greeted by a bearded figure in an apron, who
introduced himself as Bob.

I held out my hand for him to shake because I thought this was
what you are supposed to do. But somehow he didn't seem to see it,
though a moment later he glanced down at the vacant place where
it had just been poised. This weird performance reminded me of a
clip I had seen of President Kennedy ignoring the proffered hand
of CIA director Allen Dulles in exactly the same way. Which social
error had I made this time? Maybe like me, Bob disliked shaking
hands. Was that it? It remains a mystery, though I am used to social
stumbles like this.

Bob struck me as the kind of man who insists on sleeves being
folded not rolled. He brought me out the maquettes: exquisite
small-scale replicas of the proposed signs. I washed my hands with

the alcohol gel I had brought along for the purpose, and lifting the top off the large Solander box, I folded back the first sheet of tissue paper. I could feel my heart pumping faster than usual. The mock-ups had been done on 'fine fashion board' supplied by Geliot Whitman Ltd, a family-run supplier of design materials at '16A Herschell Road, Brockley Rise, London S. E. 23. Telephone FORest Hill 9262 (8 lines)'. Trading since the 1940s, Geliot Whitman had been incorporated as a limited company on 24 September 1959, and had moved to the West End in the post-war boom, being finally wound up when buying off the internet became easier than a trip to Town. I know all this because I later researched the firm's history at Companies House — surely a very Aspergery thing to do, for the information was irrelevant.

Each traffic sign was a perfect miniature, the corner radii precisely cut with a sharp craft knife. The background blue was blackish, and the green the same. I knew that Sir Hugh Casson, Chairman of the Fine Arts Commission, had suggested a green 'as dark as old dinner jackets', and this was the sort of colour finally chosen for primary 'A' routes. The more recently made signs on UK roads use noticeably brighter blues and greens, which are also lighter in tone, such that the contrast and therefore the legibility are somewhat reduced. To me they look wrong.

The yellow, white, and black symbols, lines, and characters had been painstakingly cut from paper, and glued precisely in place onto the blue, green, and white backgrounds. The signs were finished and corrected with tiny brush strokes, visible under my pocket lens.

The white paint was still crisp and bright, though the white paper had faded, leaving slightly yellow some of the paper-cutout 'holes' or so-called 'closed counters' in such characters as the Os, Ps, and zeroes.

Sliding my finger sideways across the boards I could feel the characters, arrows, and diagrammatic roads sitting proud. Everything was crisp, perfect to the width of a hair except for the board showing Dunstable and Luton, where there was an obvious paint-and-knife correction to the interior of the zero of 'A 505'. The hole had been cut five millimetres too far north — I measured it with the library ruler. Goodness knows how that mistake was made but the correction was scrupulous.

Jock Kinneir and Margaret Calvert had made these miniature likenesses with their own fingers: every mark and every cut. When these beautiful boards were bright and new, I was at school being told by a nun how infantile it was of me to pull the bobbles off my jumper.

After perusing the collection I carefully replaced the tissue sheets between the boards and closed the box. I felt as if I had been handling the Crown Jewels so I went up the road to decompress in Ye Olde Cheshire Cheese. There was a crackling fire in the grate and a young man in an expensive-looking suit was saying into his phone, 'I'm actually below target.' I got into conversation with a fellow who said he worked in advertising. I showed him a bar trick and discussed my ideas about the decline in the quality of advertising copywriting since the seventies. 'You have a half-and-half brain,' he said. 'Half analytic, half creative: exactly the right mind to work in advertising.'

★

Arriving at the family party, which had been arranged for my parents, I was able, for the first time since my diagnosis, to cast an eye around my relations, with autism in mind. My siblings were there as well as my mother and father, along with some of my nephews and nieces. I had rehearsed people's names before we arrived, even those I had known for years, as it is not only faces that throw me. My dad has always had the same problem, confusing the names of his children. He often calls me Paul.

He was, as usual, charming, if a bit odd, smartly turned out but with a quirky pair of trousers on. Though several of my mother's friends had been invited, none of the guests was a friend of my father's. As far as I know he has no friends, and as far as I remember he never has had. He seems happier alone with his nose in a book. He made me a charming apology recently for not introducing me and my brother, as youths, 'to the world of men'. This was an entirely unnecessary apology, since I now understood the reason for his distance from pubs, sport, dirty jokes, and so on. Moreover, I never wanted any such induction.

A memory sprang up from the Polaroid-tinted 1970s. My father had received a letter from the Salvation Army Tracing Service. His mother, whom he had not seen for years, was trying to find him. Dressed in shirt and slacks, with a copy of *The Acquisitive Society* in his hand, he told me tersely what the letter meant, before exclaiming, 'Bloody nerve!' and throwing it into the fire. He never heard from his mother again. Decades later, his sister made tentative contact and he replied, agreeing to meet her only so long as she could assure him that their mother was dead. When I saw my long-lost aunt she looked like a twin of my sister Esther. My dad and his sister met once or twice but for whatever reason the flame guttered out.

My brother Paul was at the party, as hilarious and odd as ever. He told me he had started to play the theorbo, a kind of long-necked lute taller than a man. He mentioned the beginnings of arthritis in his middle finger, but said that playing helped. My three sisters were there: Esther, the music teacher, was her usual brisk self, and Rebecca the Christmas baby, who had gone on to develop anxiety in lifts and on the Underground. She has taken on the role of the person who looks after everyone. My youngest sister Ruth — the only one of us seemingly untouched by Asperger's — was circulating: measured and normal. She has some high-powered job in a London art gallery.

Talking to a percussionist cousin was my son Jake, now a musician. He mentioned to me that he was finding the party hard because, 'I adopt a different personality for everyone I know and in a group of people I'm not sure who to be. I don't know who I am.' I said I knew exactly how he felt: a different mask for every situation. Jake had been to music college but, like me, had found the authoritarian and social demands almost unendurable. I recalled that my father had, himself, been unable to stand university and had left abruptly. Had we all been unlucky or did the thread of genetic non-reciprocal non-conformity run through the three of us? Were we a recusant family in more ways than one?

'There's something different about Dad,' Jake told Lea. 'He's never at ease.'

Life as the child of an Asperger can be hard. A parent who demands silence or has a meltdown if the toothpaste, or an ornament, is moved from its proper place will fill the house with dread. Now that I understand myself better I try to moderate my rules and unvarying routines but my strangeness is clear to those who know me best. As Jake had grown I had become more physically distant from him. 'Why can't you hug me, Dad?' he asked. I did not know the answer to this question, except to say that it might be a sensory problem or that I find hugging adults emotionally alarming. This is hard on Jake, but it's also hard on me. Thankfully he is much better at hugging people than I am.

Jake had taken the autism quotient test of his own accord and had scored 29, a number at the low end of the Asperger's range. He told me that, though different from me in many ways, he realises that he has always had autistic traits. Like me he was a late developer, anxious, solitary, and extraordinarily emotional under a mask of calm. Unlike me, he spends hour after hour concentrating on music.

He spoke about my mother, who was surrounded by her teenage grandchildren. 'There's nothing behind what Grandma says,' he told me. 'She just says what she thinks. I like that. It makes her easy to talk to.' If ever there was a piece of advice to people who were going to talk to an Asperger, this was it: 'Say what you mean and mean what you say.' But was my mother's saying what she meant down to ordinary straightforwardness, or was there more to it than that?

She introduced me to an aunt, who told me, 'I envied you when you were a boy: you always said exactly what you thought.' What is it with this plain speaking?

I met some cousins I hadn't seen since childhood: Sue, a librarian at Oxford University, told me she dreamt about the systemising aspects of her work: a world of rules and Dewey numbers. Her brother — my cousin Alexander — could not be at the party because he is a non-speaking, severely epileptic autistic man who needs round-the-clock care.

As the picture of autism comes better into focus, the number of girls and women on the spectrum continues to go up. Female Aspergers tend to internalise things more than men and boys, and appear better at camouflaging their true selves and fitting in. They might also express their condition by exerting rigid control over their eating. In fact, the Eating Disorder Service of the South London and Maudsley NHS Foundation Trust believes that more than a third of its patients are autistic. Further research is obviously needed into this newly emerging and vital area.

It is said that such differences in the way male and female autistics present their condition have led to delays in diagnosis. Female participants in the Cambridge 'camouflaging' study reported that parents, teachers, and professionals were disinclined to make or accept a diagnosis of autism in girls and women. A lot of work is being done to get a better idea of the ratio of female to male autistics, and it is clear that there are many more female Aspergers out there than was once thought. But as with other enduring mysteries of this condition, the picture is still not sharp.

What is clear is that no longer can autism be seen as a severe, rare, and exclusively masculine disorder. Instead of a categorically distinct condition, associated with intellectual impairments, epilepsy, and delayed language development, it is now recognised as a common way of being which presents itself in girls and women as well as in boys and men, but in different ways for each sex. It ranges in its presentation from severe to slight, blending at its slighter end into ordinary eccentricity. In the upper part of the range it is often linked with good or above average intelligence of a peculiarly focused sort and is part of the diverse picture of normal human variation, bringing with it not only a variety of special difficulties but also particular strengths and skills.

As I wandered around the party, deliberately engaging people in conversation, I spotted autistic signs among my nephews and nieces: profound dyslexia and high emotionality here, remoteness or isolation there, severe anxiety, marked food faddishness, and shut-offness in other places. There really was a lot of it about. What I also noticed was the kindness of siblings and parents in helping those who were having a hard time of it.

Lea was laughing her social laugh and being talkative in her charmingly forthright American way. A laugh is almost the first noise she makes on meeting a new person — whether it is a shop assistant, a new colleague, or a friend. She is not laughing because anything is especially funny. It is a social noise, and people respond warmly to this gregarious, open cheer. In his biography of Paul Dirac, the plainly autistic theoretical physicist, Graham Farmelo says that Simon Baron-Cohen had mentioned to him the high proportion of autistic men who establish firm and happy marriages with foreign women. Baron-Cohen was unaware that the English Dirac had been married for almost half a century to an unceasingly talkative, exceptionally empathic Hungarian wife. When I mentioned to Lea that, like me, Dirac had married his antiparticle she laughed in recognition. 'Yes,' she said, 'and I thought I was just marrying an eccentric Englishman.'

This was the first family party I had been to since my diagnosis. I was my usual slightly distant and 'aloof' self, but this time I understood more, and was able to recognise my feelings, to interpret them, and to moderate my awkward inwardness — at least a little. I managed to say hello to everybody, I did not drink too much, and I smiled more than usual. I was no longer a complete stranger in my own country. I now had a guidebook. I am learning to speak the language, though still with an accent, which gets stronger if I am tired, especially anxious, or overstimulated.

One way in which an assessment, or diagnosis, or 'label' can help an autistic person is to allow him to moderate his behaviour. I try hard to quell my tendency to be critical of everything and to let my discontents be my secrets. I don't know if anybody at the party noticed, but I was pleased with my performance. Anyway, it was a start.

We were driven home by a friend, who was telling us about an occasion when his horse rolled on top of him, doing him some damage. I felt Lea banging me in the ribs with her elbow. Afterwards she explained: 'You interrupted David with your own story before he had finished. *As usual*. And you were speaking much too loudly again.' Plainly I must try harder.

Autumn was about, and the carotenes were causing a red and purple riot in the leaves. Prickly horse chestnuts fell from their twigs, their splitting pulp exposing conkers like gorillas' eyes. The weather had been dry and hot for weeks but now it was getting close. Giant thunderheads towered above the South Downs. A grumbling storm was approaching.

I thought about other people from my past. 'Auntie' Mary, who had taken it well when I shouted bugger through the library letter flap, was living in a nursing home; 'Uncle' David, who in his rainy shed had first interested me in magic, had long since gone to his reward; Jon, my oldest friend, had retired from teaching and now painted all day in his house in Wales, or in the hills beyond. We spoke on the telephone most weeks. Strawberry blonde Alice I knew was married with three grown-up children; Anthony had retired from his job as a postman and spent his days painting or making prints. He told me that one day before his retirement he had delivered a packet to the offices of a Soho advertising agency. The boss, a tall dark man, stepped out to sign for it. 'Guess who it was,' said Anthony. I had no idea. 'Bob Scotland!' — the student who had painted a four-foot wide black stripe over everybody's marks in the futile first-year exercise at the university, a quarter of a century earlier.

'Did you speak to him?' I asked.

'I don't think he recognised me,' said Anthony.

I remembered Bob in the all-male Starley Hall, striding across the muddy quad from the refectory, two breakfasts in his arms — one for the young woman he was quite illegally keeping in his room, and servicing nightly. Everyone knew but he didn't care. Though I disapproved of the rule breaking, I took my hat off to his flouting of mere authority. Plumbing the bowels of the World Wide Web I tried to pin down Anthony's recollection but could find no reference to Bob Scotland.

The story was different for Bob Strange, the student who had shown me the pamphlet about the stigmatic Padre Pio. I found an internet photograph of him in 0.37 seconds. He was perched on top of a scaffold tower, holding a palette bigger than a dustbin lid, painting a religious mural in a Catholic church.

My editor Dan was no longer a scampish-schoolboy but juggled millions as the UK head of a multinational publishing company. Royalties were still coming in for the book I had written for him more than a decade before.

Leo Kanner and Hans Asperger had died in the eighties, within a year of each other. But there was a shock in store. In her 2018 book *Asperger's Children*, historian Edith Sheffer confirmed suggestions that Asperger's relationship with the Nazis had been much closer than generally thought. Using documents from the time, Sheffer made a persuasive case that, although Asperger had protected children he considered intelligent, he knowingly referred others to a 'child euthanasia' clinic in Vienna. This is an appalling revelation, but it is one which I maintain does nothing to detract from the usefulness of his work on the syndrome that has borne his name since Lorna Wing explained it to the world. Others disagree strongly with my view.

Jock Kinnear, co-designer of those beautifully clear and powerful traffic signs, died in 1994, but, at the time of writing, Margaret Calvert is still alive. Her water-clear slab serif character set has been introduced in a gigantic size on the platforms of Tyne and Wear Metro: a joyful and vividly effective bit of design. She was also type and pictogram consultant for the Moscow Metro's superb new signage system. One day my friend Louise, who runs a gallery, told me that she had commissioned Calvert to make a print of her *Woman at Work* painting in a limited edition of twenty-five. *Woman at Work* resembles her famous men at work sign, but instead of the silhouette of a male labourer 'wrestling with a big umbrella' it features a digging woman. I knew at once that I must have one of these so I crossed Louise's palm with silver. Quite a lot of silver. When the print arrived it was accompanied, to my delight, by a charming letter in Calvert's own hand, addressed 'Dear Tom' and signed simply 'Margaret'. Louise had told her of my lifelong enthusiasm. I felt like a teenage girl getting a personal note from the pop star over whom she has been mooning for years. I don't think I have ever received such a giddying letter.

★

It was unseasonably muggy. People in roadside cafés wafted themselves with menus as I walked over the bridge to check on the progress of the new flood defences along the river. The navvies were pouring bottled water over their heads as a vast hydraulic driver vibrated miles of sheet piling into the riverbed.

Tracking the progress of civil engineering projects fills me with geekish glee. I stand and watch, like a supervisor, for minutes at a time. I seem to have turned into the man at parties I used to warn myself about. Over the years I have assembled a large album of photographs of pylons, canal bridges, and a few rather nice gridded drain covers. As a boy I was fascinated by gyroscopes and since that time I have put together a collection of small spinning tops. Whenever I see one I like I buy it, and it adds a pinch of amused enjoyment to my odd hobby to have learnt of the autistic fascination for spinning things.

I am now eight years older than my maternal grandfather was when he died. No longer the haunted schoolboy, 'lost in a world of his own', I have become the grey-snouted man who is offered a seat on the Tube.

If there were a button I could press to abolish my Asperger's syndrome, its pains, but also its quirky gifts, would I press it? Would I? There is a famous quote from Rilke: 'Don't take away my devils, for my angels might flee too', but I wonder if the devils of anguish, confusion, exhaustion, and constant loneliness are really worth the angels. I asked my juggling friend Gary if he would press the button. He said no.

The web of our lives is of mingled yarn, good and ill together, and circumstances unfold so capriciously, so unjustly, that our happiness seems to have been no part of the plan. Some see this through the window of faith, others through the window of doubt, but we are all, in the end, obliged to make our own meaning.

★

Shortly before this book was due to go to print, I decided to let my family know about my diagnosis. I rang my sister Ruth first.

'Oh,' she said, 'Asperger's. Thanks for telling me. It's hardly surprising, of course; Dad's dad was autistic.'

'You what?' I said. I felt as if I'd been hit.

'Yes, didn't you know? It's one of the reasons Granddad left his family so abruptly.'

My mouth was hanging open; I was stunned. Why on earth had nobody ever mentioned this vital family fact? How different might things have been had I known?

★

The rain had begun falling in big drops, which spread into ink blots on the paving stones. The tang of petrichor filled the air, and then ozone as a sudden flash of lightning split the sky, attended by a thunderclap so loud it made a yellow dog and her owner jump. I darted into a café as the rain became a drumming torrent, pouring down windows, bouncing off canopies and pavements, and sweeping great beavers' lodges of leaves and litter along the gutters, deep down into the drains. The thirsty earth swallowed the lot.

Then, as quickly as it had started, the deluge stopped; people came out from under dripping awnings, shaking umbrellas. Away to the north, between the storm clouds and the distant hills, blue-grey smears of rain were still visible. On the horizon a rainbow had appeared.

A fresh breeze was blowing up from the front, jiggling the water droplets that hung from a traffic sign. 'NEW ROAD LAYOUT AHEAD' it announced. On a low wall, a bird was fluttering spray from its plumage and nearby a young mother was laughing loudly as her child splashed in the gullies. There is only one happiness: to love and be loved. As I stepped out of the café the sudden sun caught me full in the face, stretching my shadow along the shining pavement behind me. Dodging the puddles I crossed the car park, heading for the bridge that would take me over the river, across the water, towards home.

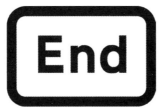

Acknowledgements

It takes more than one person to make a book and I would like to thank the following people who helped me with this one.

I am especially grateful to Scribe's Publisher-at-Large Philip Gwyn Jones, who commissioned the title and remained my cheerful and astute companion throughout the journey, guiding me gently this way and that. He indulged my foibles, made useful suggestions, and, with the kindness, as it were, of a much-loved family doctor, strangled at birth my bad ideas, my tendency to go on a bit, and my foul-ups with Latin infinitives. Molly Slight, who took up the editorial scalpel, was likewise a model of sharp-witted good sense all the way, euthanising some accidentally offensive passages, and a rash of pointless commas. She also saved me from embarrassment by alerting me to several major goofs. Any remaining blunders are my own. Scribe's Laura Thomas also deserves my thanks. She is the designer of many stylish books, and made this one look as good as it does.

Praise is due, as always, to my ever-smiling agent Laura Morris, who supplied steadfast encouragement through thick and thin, driven by an iron-hard conviction that this book should see the light, and that the game really was worth the candle.

Linguist David Crystal generously answered my early queries about the propriety of coining the term 'Asperger', which he thought was 'okay', though he warned me that my newly minted adjective 'Aspergic' might be confused with an aspirin product of a similar name. He pointed me towards 'Aspergerian', but I objected that the Aspergerians were surely creatures from *Star Trek* or *Doctor Who*.

I salute those who read bits of this book in draft and gave me their opinions, expert and otherwise. From the start, the National Autistic Society's Autism Access Specialist Chris Pike, and Culture and Features Media Relations Manager Louisa Mullan, went out of their way to be helpful. The same was true of Sarah Hendrickx, who, after formally identifying me as being on the autism spectrum, proved a fount of information and never tired of answering my questions.

West Sussex libraries and the British Library were obliging in tracking down various books, some of them rather out of the way. Of general interest I particularly recommend Adam Feinstein's definitive *A History of Autism: conversations with the pioneers* (Wiley-Blackwell, 2010) and Steve Silberman's *NeuroTribes: the legacy of autism and how to think smarter about people who think differently* (Allen & Unwin, 2015), both of which I turned to from time to time.

When I wanted to examine Jock Kinneir and Margaret Calvert's original road sign maquettes the staff of St Bride Library took pains to make things easy for me, and were only too keen to expand on their curatorial history. I likewise thank Anna Kinneir of the Jock

Kinneir Library for some fascinating conversations, and Margaret Calvert, who troubled to write me a charming letter.

The road traffic signs which appear at the head of chapters and on the front cover of this book are Crown copyright; I am grateful for permission to use them. I am obliged also to the Autism Research Centre at the University of Cambridge for responding positively to my request to reproduce the Autism-Spectrum Quotient, on page 93, and the scatter plot, on page 104. The ARC is an excellent resource for anybody interested in reading some of the most illuminating and useful recent research into the autism spectrum, including Asperger's syndrome. Their policy of using language 'understanded of the people' means that any moderately intelligent person can get to grips with their work.

I am particularly grateful to my friends and family for their forbearance over the years, as I am not the easiest chap to get along with. I decided that almost all of those I mention in the book would prefer to remain unidentified, so the names I have given them are mostly not their own.

Finally, of course, I thank 'Lea': the most wonderfully patient, kind, ebullient, protective, understanding, humorous, apt, and lovely non-autistic woman any Asperger could hope for. Without her I seriously do not know what would have become of me.